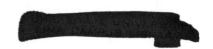

Fundamentals of
Medicinal Chemistry

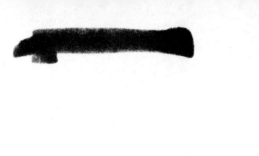

Fundamentals of Medicinal Chemistry

Gareth Thomas

University of Portsmouth, UK

WILEY

Copyright © 2003 John Wiley & Sons Ltd,
The Atrium, Southern Gate, Chichester,
West Sussex PO19 8SQ, England

Telephone   (+44) 1243 779777

Email (for orders and customer service enquiries): cs-books@wiley.co.uk
Visit our Home Page on www.wileyeurope.com or www.wiley.com

Reprinted August 2004

Other Wiley Editorial Offices

John Wiley & Sons Inc., 111 River Street, Hoboken, NJ 07030, USA

Jossey-Bass, 989 Market Street, San Francisco, CA 94103-1741, USA

Wiley-VCH Verlag GmbH, Boschstr. 12, D-69469 Weinheim, Germany

John Wiley & Sons Australia Ltd, 33 Park Road, Milton, Queensland 4064, Australia

John Wiley & Sons (Asia) Pte Ltd, 2 Clementi Loop #02-01, Jin Xing Distripark, Singapore 129809

John Wiley & Sons Canada Ltd, 22 Worcester Road, Etobicoke, Ontario, Canada M9W 1L1

Library of Congress Cataloging-in-Publication Data

Thomas, Gareth, Dr.
    Fundamentals of medicinal chemistry / Gareth Thomas.
    p. cm
Includes bibliographical references and index.
    ISBN 0-470-84306-3 (cloth : alk. paper)   ISBN 0-470-84307-1 (paper : alk. paper)
1. Pharmaceutical chemistry. I. Title
    RS403.T446 2003
    615'.19 — — dc21   2003014218

British Library Cataloguing in Publication Data

A catalogue record for this book is available from the British Library

ISBN 0-470-84306-3 (Hardback)
ISBN 0-470-84307-1 (Paperback)

Typeset in 11/14 Times by Kolam Information Services Pvt. Ltd, Pondicherry, India.
Printed and bound in Great Britain by Antony Rowe Ltd, Chippenham, Wiltshire.
This book is printed on acid-free paper responsibly manufactured from sustainable forestry in which at least two trees are planted for each one used for paper production.

Contents

Preface

This book is written for second, and subsequent year undergraduates studying for degrees in medicinal chemistry, pharmaceutical chemistry, pharmacy, pharmacology and other related degrees. It is also intended for students whose degree courses contain a limited reference to medicinal chemistry. The text assumes that the reader has a knowledge of chemistry at level one of a university life sciences degree. The text discusses the fundamental chemical principles used for drug discovery and design. A knowledge of physiology and biology is advantageous but not essential. Appropriate relevant physiology and biology is outlined in the appendices.

Chapter 1 gives a brief review of the structures and nomenclature of the more common classes of naturally occurring compounds found in biological organisms. It is included for undergraduates who have little or no background knowledge of natural product chemistry. For students who have studied natural product chemistry it may be used as either a revision or a reference chapter. Chapter 2 attempts to give an overview of medicinal chemistry. The basic approaches used to discover and design drugs are outlined in Chapters 3–6 inclusive. Chapter 7 is intended to give the reader a taste of main line medicinal chemistry. It illustrates some of the strategies used, often within the approaches outlined in previous chapters, to design new drugs. For a more encyclopedic coverage of the discovery and design of drugs for specific conditions, the reader is referred to appropriate texts such as some of those given under *Medicinal Chemistry* in the *Selected Further Reading* section at the end of this book. Chapters 8 and 9 describe the pharmacokinetics and metabolism respectively of drugs and their effect on drug design. Chapter 10 attempts to give an introductory overview of an area that is one of the principal objectives of the medicinal chemist. For a more in depth discussion, the reader is referred to the many specialized texts that are available on organic synthesis. Drug development from the research stage to marketing the final product is briefly outlined in Chapter 11.

The approach to medicinal chemistry is kept as simple as possible. The text is supported by a set of questions at the end of each chapter. Answers, sometimes in the form of references to sections of the book, are listed separately. A list of recommended further reading, classified according to subject, is also included.

Gareth Thomas

Acknowledgements

I wish to thank all my colleagues, past and present without, whose help this book would have not been written. In particular, I would like to thank Dr. S Arkle for access to his lecture notes and Dr. J Wong for his unstinted help and advice, Dr. J Brown for again acting as a living pharmacology dictionary, Dr. P Cox for the molecular model diagrams and his patience in explaining to me the intricacies of molecular modelling and Mr. A Barrow and Dr. D Brimage for the library searches they conducted. I wish also to thank the following friends and colleagues for proof-reading chapters and supplying information: Dr. L Adams, Dr. C Alexander, Dr. L Banting, Dr. D Brown, Dr. S Campbell, Dr. B Carpenter, Mr. P Clark, Dr. P Howard, Dr. A Hunt, Mrs. W Jones, Dr. T Mason, Dr. J Mills, Dr. T Nevell, Dr. M Norris, Dr. J Smart, Professor D Thurston, Dr. G White and Mr. S Wills.

Finally, I would like to thank my wife for her support whilst I was writing the text.

Abbreviations

A	Adenine
Abe	Abequose
ACE	Angiotensin-converting enzyme
ACh	Acetyl choline
ADME	Absorption, distribution, metabolism and elimination
ADR	Adverse drug reaction
Ala	Alanine
Arg	Arginine
Asp	Aspartate
ATP	Deoxyadenosine triphosphate
dATP	Adenosine triphosphate
AUC	Area under the curve
C	Cytosine
CNS	Central nervous system
CoA	Coenzyme A
CYP-450	Cytochrome P-450 family
Cys	Cysteine
d.e.	Diastereoisometric excess
DHF	Dihydrofolic acid
DHFR	Dihydrofolate reductase
DMPK	Drug metabolism and pharmacokinetics
DNA	Deoxyribonucleic acid
EC	Enzyme commission
e.e.	Enantiomeric excess
ELF	Effluent load factor
EMEA	European medicines evaluation agency
EPC	European Patent Convention
EPO	European Patent Office
E_s	Taft steric parameter

FDA	Food and drugs administration
FMO	Flavin monoxygenase
FGI	Functional group interconversion
Fmoc,	9-Fluorenylmethoxychloroformyl group
FdUMP	5-fluoro-2′-deoxyuridyline monophosphate
FUdRP	5-fluoro-2′-deoxyuridylic acid
G	Guanine
GABA	γ-Aminobutyric acid
GI	Gastrointestinal tract
Gln	Glutamine
Glu	Glutamatic acid
Gly	Glycine
GSH	Glutathione
Hb,	Haemoglobin
HbS	Sickel cell haemoglobin
His	Histidine
HIV	Human immunodeficiency disease
hnRNA	Heterogeneous nuclear RNA
Ile	Isoleucine
IV	Intravenous injection
IM	Intramuscular injection
KDO	2-Keto-3-deoxyoctanoate
LDA	Lithium diisopropylamide
LDH	Lactose dehydrogenase
Leu	Leucine
Lys	Lysine
mACh	Muscarinic cholinergic receptor
MA(A)	Market authorisation (application)
MCA	Medical control agency
Met	Methionine
Moz	4-Methoxybenzyloxychloroformyl group
MR	Molar refractivity
mRNA	messenger RNA
nACh	Nicotinic cholinergic receptor
NAD^+	Nicotinamide adenine dinucleotide (oxidised form)
NADH	Nicotinamide adenine dinucleotide (reduced form)

NADP$^+$ Nicotinamide dinucleotide phosphate (oxidised form)
NADPH   Nicotinamide dinucleotide phosphate (reduced form)
NAG   β-N-Acetylglucosamine
NAM   β-N-Acetylmuramic acid

ONs   Sequence defined oligonucleotides

P-450   Cytochrome P-450 oxidases
PABA p-Aminobenzoic acid
PCT   Paten Cooperation Treaty
PG   Prostaglandin
Phe   Phenylalanine
PO   Per oral (by mouth)
pre-mRNA   Premessenger RNA
Pro   Proline
ptRNA   Primary transcript RNA

QSAR   Quantitative structural-activity relationships

RNA   Ribonucleic acid

SAM S-Adenosylmethionine
SAR   *See* Structural-activity relationships
Ser   Serine
SIN-1   3-Morpholino-sydnomine

T   Thymine
THF   Tetrahydrofolic acid
Thr   Threonine
dTMP   Deoxythymidylate-5′-monophosphate
tRNA   transfer RNA
Try   Tyrosine

U   Uracil
UDP   Uridine diphosphate
UDPGA   Uridine diphosphate glucuronic acid
dUMP   Deoxyuridylate-5′-monophosphate
UdRP   Deoxyuridylic acid

Val   Valine

1 Biological Molecules

1.1 Introduction

Chemical compounds and metallic ions are the basic building blocks of all biological structures and processes that are the basis of life as we know it. Some of these naturally occuring compounds and ions (**endogenous species**) are present only in very small amounts in specific regions of the body, whilst others, such as peptides, proteins, carbohydrates, lipids and nucleic acids, are found in all parts of the body. A basic knowledge of the nomenclature and structures of these more common endogenous classes of biological molecules is essential to understanding medicinal chemistry. This chapter introduces these topics in an attempt to provide for those readers who do not have this background knowledge.

The structures of biologically active molecules usually contain more than one type of functional group. This means that the properties of these molecules are a mixture of those of each of the functional groups present plus properties characteristic of the compound. The latter are frequently due to the interaction of adjacent functional groups and/or the influence of a functional group on the carbon–hydrogen skeleton of the compound. This often involves the electronic activation of C–H bonds by adjacent functional groups.

1.2 Amino acids

1.2.1 Introduction

Simple amino acids are the basic building blocks of proteins. Their structures contain both an amino group, usually a primary amine, and a carboxylic acid. The relative positions of these groups vary, but for most naturally occurring

Fundamentals of Medicinal Chemistry, Edited by Gareth Thomas
© 2003 John Wiley & Sons, Ltd
ISBN 0 470 84306 3 (Hbk), ISBN 0 470 84307 1 (pbk)

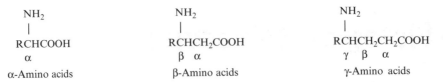

Figure 1.1 The general structural formulae of amino acids. Amino acids may be classified as α, β, γ ....etc. depending on the relative positions of the amine and carboxylic acid groups. α-Amino acids are the most common naturally occuring amino acids

compounds the amino group is attached to the same carbon as the carboxylic acid (Figure 1.1).

The structures of amino acids can also contain other functional groups besides the amine and carboxylic acid groups (Table 1.1). Methionine, for example, contains a sulphide group, whilst serine has a primary alcohol group.

Table 1.1 Examples of the names and structures of amino acids

Amino acid	Name	Symbol/letter		$pI(25°)$
$CH_3CH_2(NH_2)COOH$	Alanine	Ala	A	6.0
$NH_2\text{-}\overset{\overset{NH}{\|\|}}{C}\text{-}NHCH_2CH_2CH_2CH(NH_2)COOH$	Arginine	Arg	R	10.8
$NH_2COCH_2CH(NH_2)COOH$	Asparagine	Asn	N	5.4
$HOOCCH_2CH(NH_2)COOH$	Aspartic acid	Asp	D	3.0
$HOOCCH_2CH_2CH(NH_2)COOH$	Glutamic acid	Glu	E	3.2
$H_2NCOCH_2CH_2CH(NH_2)COOH$	Glutamine	Gln	Q	5.7
$CH_2(NH_2)COOH$	Glycine	Gly	G	6.0
$CH_2CH(NH_2)COOH$ (imidazole)	Histidine	His	H	7.6
$\overset{\overset{CH_3}{\|}}{CH_3CH_2CHCH(NH_2)COOH}$	Isoleucine	Ile	I	6.0
$\overset{\overset{CH_3}{\|}}{CH_3CHCH_2CH(NH_2)COOH}$	Leucine	Leu	L	5.9
$H_2NCH_2CH_2CH_2CH_2CH(NH_2)COOH$	Lysine	Lys	K	9.7
$CH_3SCH_2CH_2CH(NH_2)COOH$	Methionine	Met	M	5.7
$PhCH_2CH(NH_2)COOH$	Phenylalanine	Phe	F	5.5
$COOH$ (pyrrolidine, NH)	Proline	Pro	P	6.3
$CH_2OHCH(NH_2)COOH$	Serine	Ser	S	5.7
$\overset{\overset{CH_3}{\|}}{CH_3CHCH(NH_2)COOH}$	Valine	Val	V	6.0

The nature of the side chains of amino acids determines the hydrophobic (water hating) and hydrophilic (water loving) nature of the amino acid. Amino acids with hydrophobic side chains will be less soluble in water than those with hydrophilic side chains. The hydrophobic/hydrophilic nature of the side chains of amino acids has a considerable influence on the conformation adopted by a peptide or protein in aqueous solution. Furthermore, the hydrophobic/hydrophilic balance of the groups in a molecule will have a considerable effect on the ease of its passage through membranes (Appendix 5).

1.2.2 Structure

All solid amino acids exist as dipolar ions known as zwitterions (Figure 1.2(a)). In aqueous solution the structure of amino acids are dependent on the pH of the solution (Figure 1.2(b)). The pH at which an aqueous solution of an amino acid is electrically neutral is known as the **isoelectric point (pI)** of the amino acid (Table 1.1). Isoelectric point values vary with temperature. They are used in the design of electrophoretic and chromatographic analytical methods for amino acids.

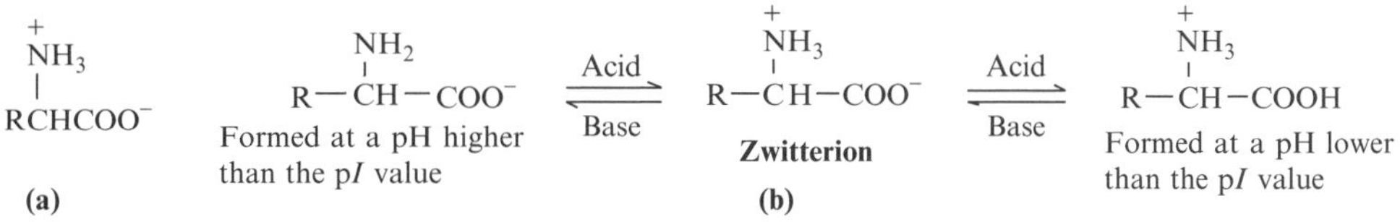

Figure 1.2 (a) The general structural formula of the zwitterions of amino acids. (b) The structures of amino acids in acidic and basic aqueous solutions

1.2.3 Nomenclature

Amino acids are normally known by their trivial names (Table 1.1). In peptide and protein structures their structures are indicated by either three letter groups or single letters (Table 1.1, and Figure 1.7). Amino acids such as ornithine and citrulline, which are not found in naturally occuring peptides and proteins, do not have an allocated three or single letter code (Figure 1.3).

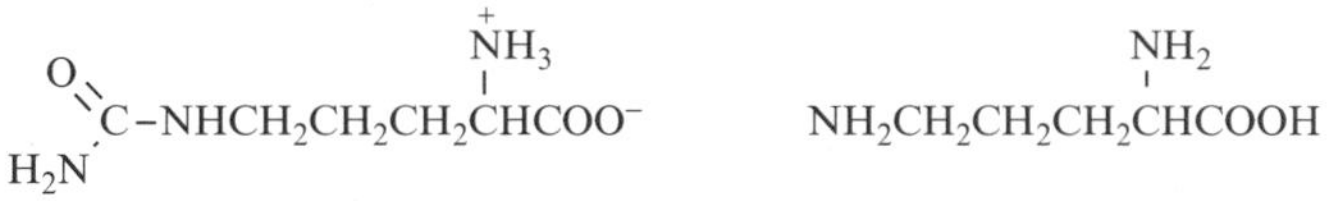

Figure 1.3 Ornithine and citrulline

Most amino acids, with the notable exception of glycine, are optically active. Their configurations are usually indicated by the D/L system (Figure 1.4) rather than the R/S system. Most naturally occuring amino acids have an L configuration but there are some important exceptions. For example, some bacteria also possess D-amino acids. This is important in the development of some antibacterial drugs.

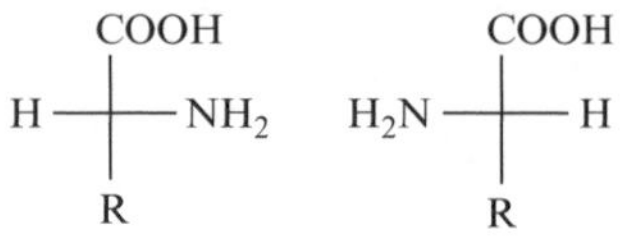

$$
\begin{array}{cc}
\text{COOH} & \text{COOH} \\
H -\!\!\!\!\mid\!\!\!\!- NH_2 & H_2N -\!\!\!\!\mid\!\!\!\!- H \\
R & R \\
\text{D series} & \text{L series}
\end{array}
$$

Figure 1.4 The D/L configurations of amino acids. Note that the carboxylic acid group must be drawn at the top and the R group at the bottom of the Fischer projection. Stereogenetic centres in the R group do not affect the D/L assignment

1.3 Peptides and proteins

Peptides and proteins have a wide variety of roles in the human body (Table 1.2). They consist of amino acid residues linked together by **amide functional groups** (Figure 1.5(a)), which in peptides and proteins are referred to as **peptide links** (Figure 1.5(c)). The amide group has a rigid flat structure. The lone pair of its nitrogen atom is able to interact with the π electrons of the carbonyl group.

Table 1.2 Examples of some of the biological functions of proteins

Function	Notes
Structural	These proteins provide strength and elasticity to, for example, bone (collagen), hair (α-keratins) and connective tissue (elastin).
Enzymes	This is the largest class of proteins. Almost all steps in biological reactions are catalysed by enzymes.
Regulatory	These are proteins that control the physiological activity of other proteins. Insulin, for example, regulates glucose metabolism in mammals.
Transport	These transport specific compounds from one part of the body to another haemoglobin transports carbon dioxide too and oxygen from the lungs. Cell membranes contain proteins that are responsible for the transport of species from one side of the membrane to the other.
Storage	These provide a store of substances required by the body. For example, the protein ferritin acts as an iron store for the body.
Protective	These proteins that protect the body. Some form part of the bodies immune system defending the body against foreign molecules and bacteria. Others, such as the blood clotting agents thrombin and fibrinogen, prevent loss of blood when a blood vessel is damaged.

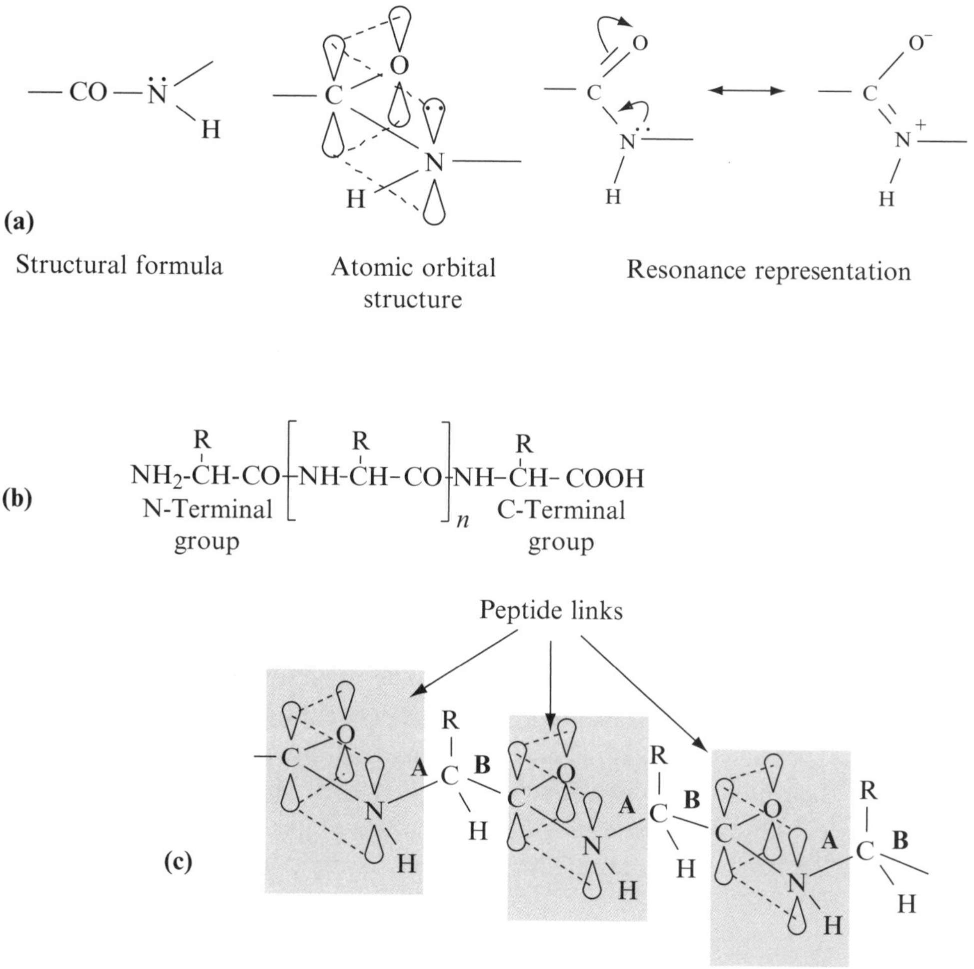

(a)

Structural formula   Atomic orbital structure   Resonance representation

(b)

$$NH_2\text{-}\overset{R}{\underset{\mid}{C}}H\text{-}CO\left[NH\text{-}\overset{R}{\underset{\mid}{C}}H\text{-}CO\right]_n NH\text{-}\overset{R}{\underset{\mid}{C}}H\text{-}COOH$$

N-Terminal group   C-Terminal group

Peptide links

(c)

Figure 1.5 (a) The structure of the amide functional group. (b) The general structure of simple peptides. (c) The peptide link is planar and has a rigid conjugated structure. Changes in conformation can occur about bonds A and B. Adapted from G Thomas, *Chemistry for Pharmacy and the Life Sciences including Pharmacology and Biomedical Science*, 1996, published by Prentice Hall, a Pearson Education Company

This electron delocalization is explained by p orbital overlap and is usually shown by the use of resonance structures (Figure 1.5(a)).

The term **peptide** is normally used for compounds that contain small numbers of amino acid residues whilst the term **polypeptide** is loosely used for larger compounds with relative molecular mass (RMM) values greater than about 500 or more. **Proteins** are more complex polypeptides with RMM values usually greater than 2000. They are classified as **simple** when their structures contain only amino acid residues and **conjugated** when other residues besides those of amino acids occur as integral parts of their structures. For example, haemoglobin is a conjugated protein because its structure contains a haem residue (Figure 1.6). These non-amino-acid residues are known as **prosthetic groups** when they are involved in the biological activity of the molecule. Conjugated proteins are classified according to the chemical nature of their non-amino-acid component. For example, glycoproteins contain a carbohydrate residue, haemoproteins a haem group and lipoproteins a lipid residue.

1.3.1   Structure

The structures of peptides and proteins are very varied. They basically consist of chains of amino acid residues (Figures 1.5(b), 1.5(c) and 1.7). These chains may be branched due to the presence of multi-basic or acidic amino acid residues in the chain (Figure 1.7(d)). In addition, bridges (cross links) may be formed between different sections of the same chain or different chains. Cysteine residues, for example, are responsible for the S–S bridges between the two peptide chains that form the structure of insulin (Figure 1.7(e)). The basic structure of peptides and proteins is twisted into a conformation (time dependent overall shape) characteristic of that peptide or protein. These conformations are dependent on both the nature of their biological environment as well as their chemical structures. The ability of peptides and proteins to carry out their biological functions is normally dependent on this conformation. Any changes to any part of the structure of a

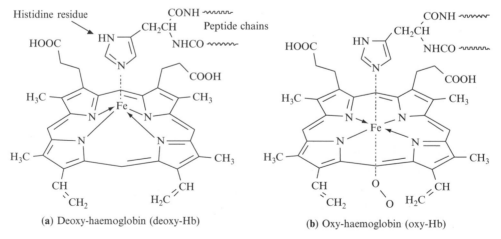

(a) Deoxy-haemoglobin (deoxy-Hb)   (b) Oxy-haemoglobin (oxy-Hb)

Figure 1.6   The structure of the haem residue in deoxy- and oxy-haemoglobins. In deoxy-Hb the bonding of the iron is pyramidal whilst in oxy-Hb it is octahedral

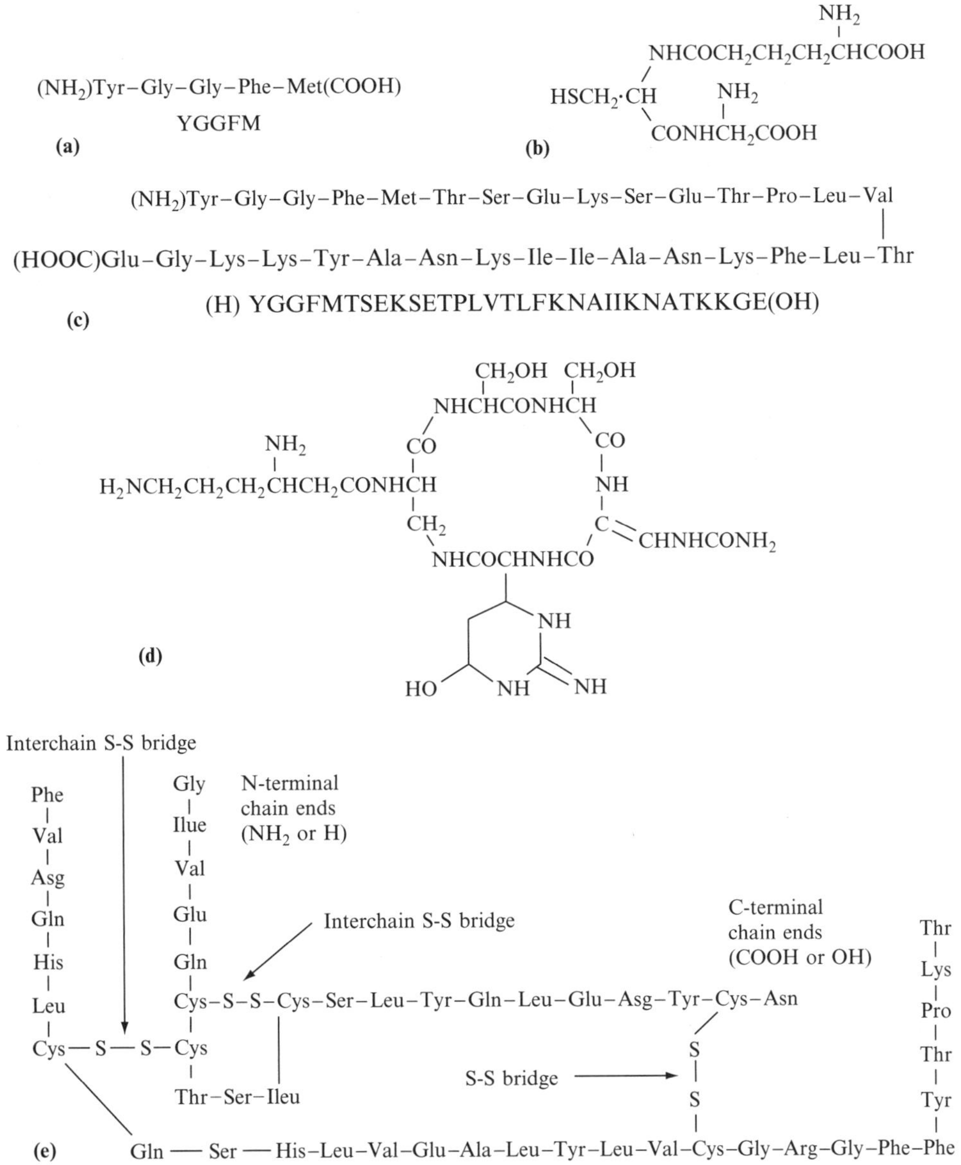

(a)

(NH$_2$)Tyr–Gly–Gly–Phe–Met(COOH)

YGGFM

(b)

$$
\begin{array}{c}
\text{NH}_2 \\
|\\
\text{NHCOCH}_2\text{CH}_2\text{CH}_2\text{CHCOOH}\\
\end{array}
$$

HSCH$_2$·CH 　 NH$_2$

CONHCH$_2$COOH

(c)

(NH$_2$)Tyr–Gly–Gly–Phe–Met–Thr–Ser–Glu–Lys–Ser–Glu–Thr–Pro–Leu–Val

(HOOC)Glu–Gly–Lys–Lys–Tyr–Ala–Asn–Lys–Ile–Ile–Ala–Asn–Lys–Phe–Leu–Thr

(H) YGGFMTSEKSETPLVTLFKNAIIKNATKKGE(OH)

(d)

CH$_2$OH CH$_2$OH

NHCHCONHCH

NH$_2$ 　 CO 　 CO

H$_2$NCH$_2$CH$_2$CH$_2$CHCH$_2$CONHCH 　 NH

CH$_2$ 　 C

NHCOCHNHCO 　 CHNHCONH$_2$

NH

HO 　 NH 　 NH

(e)

Interchain S-S bridge

Phe
|
Val
|
Asg
|
Gln
|
His
|
Leu
|
Cys — S — S — Cys

Gly
|
Ilue
|
Val
|
Glu
|
Gln
|
Cys–S–S–Cys–Ser–Leu–Tyr–Gln–Leu–Glu–Asg–Tyr–Cys–Asn
|
Thr–Ser–Ileu

N-terminal
chain ends
(NH$_2$ or H)

Interchain S-S bridge

C-terminal
chain ends
(COOH or OH)

Thr
|
Lys
|
Pro
|
Thr
|
Tyr

S
|
S

S-S bridge

Gln — Ser — His–Leu–Val–Glu–Ala–Leu–Tyr–Leu–Val–Cys–Gly–Arg–Gly–Phe–Phe

Figure 1.7 Representations of the primary structures of peptides. Two systems of abreviations are used to represent primary structures. The single letter system is used for computer programs. In both systems the N-terminus of the peptide chain is usually drawn on the left-hand side of the structure. (a) Met-enkephalin. This pentapeptide occurs in human brain tissue. (b) Glutathione, an important constituent of all cells, where it is involved in a number of biological processes. (c) β-Endorphin. This endogenous peptide has opiate activity and is believed to be produced in the body to counter pain. (d) Viomycin, a polypeptide antibiotic produced by *Streptomyces griseoverticillatus* var. *tuberacticus*. The presence of the dibasic 2,3-diaminoproanoic acid residue produces the chain branching. (e) Insulin, the hormone that is responsible for controlling glucose metabolism

peptide or protein will either change or destroy the compound's biological activity. For example, sickle-cell anaemia (Appendix 1) is caused by the replacement of a glutamine residue by a valine residue structure of haemoglobin.

Proteins are often referred to as **globular** and **fibrous proteins** according to their conformation. Globular proteins are usually soluble in water, whilst fibrous proteins are usually insoluble. The complex nature of their structures has resulted in the use of a sub-classification, sometimes referred to as **the order of protein structures**. This classification divides the structure into into primary, secondary, tertiary and quaternary orders of structures.

The **primary protein structure** of peptides and proteins is the sequence of amino acid residues in the molecule (Figure. 1.7).

Secondary protein structures are the local regular and random conformations assumed by sections of the peptide chains found in the structures of peptides and proteins. The main regular conformations found in the secondary structures of proteins are the α-helix, the β-pleated sheet and the triple helix (Figure 1.8). These and other random conformations are believed to be mainly due to intramolecular hydrogen bonding between different sections of the peptide chain.

The **tertiary protein structure** is the overall shape of the molecule. Tertiary structures are often formed by the peptide chain folding back on itself. These folded structures are stabilized by S–S bridges, hydrogen bonding, salt bridges (Figure 1.9(a)) and van der Waals' forces within the peptide chain and also with molecules in the peptide's environment. They are also influenced by hydrophobic interactions between the peptide chain and its environment. Hydrophobic interaction is thought to be mainly responsible for the folded shape of the β-peptide chain of human haemoglobin (Figure 1.9(b)). In this structure the hydrophilic groups of the peptide chain are on the outer surface of the folded structure.

Quaternary protein structures are the three dimensional protein structures formed by the noncovalent associations of a number of individual peptides and polypeptide molecules. These individual peptide and polypeptide molecules are known as subunits. They may or may not be the same. Haemoglobin, for example, consists of four subunits, two α- and two β-units held together by hydrogen bonds and salt bridges.

The structures of peptides and proteins usually contain numerous amino and carboxylic acid groups. Consequently, water soluble proteins in aqueous solution can form differently charged structures and zwitterions depending on the pH of the solution (see 1.2.2). The pH at which the latter occurs is known as the isoelectric point (pI) of the protein (Table 1.3). The nature of the charge on the structures of peptides and proteins has a considerable effect on their solubility

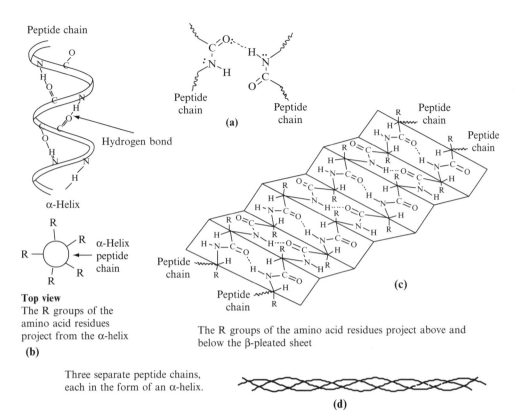

Figure 1.8 The secondary structures of proteins. (a) Hydrogen bonding between peptide links. The conjugated lone pair of the amide nitrogen atom is not available to form hydrogen bonds. (b) The α-helix. The peptide chain is largely held in this shape by intramolecular hydrogen bonds. (c) β-Pleated sheets are formed by hydrogen bonding between neighbouring peptide chains. Antiparallel β-sheets (shown) have the peptide chains running in opposite directions. Parallel β-sheet (not shown) have the peptide chains running in the same direction. Silk fibroin has a high proportion of antiparallel β-pleated sheets. (d) The triple helix in which the three peptide chains are largely held together by hydrogen bonding. For example, the basis of the structure of the fibrous protein collagen which occurs in skin, teeth and bones, consists of three chains of the polypeptide tropocollagen in the form of a triple helix. This forms a cable like structure known as a *protofibril*. Reproduced from G Thomas, *Chemistry for Pharmacy and the Life Sciences including Pharmacology and Biomedical Science*, 1996, by permission of Prentice Hall, a Pearson Education Company

and biological activity. For example, the water solubility of a protein is usually at a minimum at its isoelectric point whilst the charge on a protein may affect the ease of transport of a protein through a plasma membrane (see Appendix 5). It is also important in electrophoretic and chromatographic methods of protein analysis.

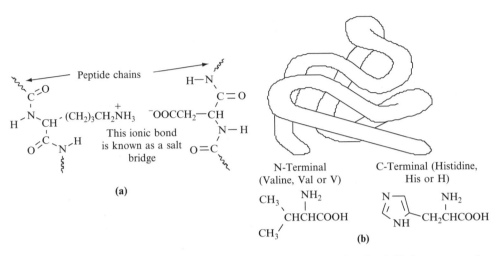

Figure 1.9 (a) A salt bridge. This is essentially an ionic bond. (b) The folded structure of a β-haemoglobin polypeptide chain. Reproduced from G Thomas, *Chemistry for Pharmacy and the Life Sciences including Pharmacology and Biomedical Science*, 1996, by permission of Prentice Hall, a Pearson Education Company

Table 1.3 Examples of the pI values of proteins (various sources)

Protein	pI (25°)	Protein	pI (25°)	Protein	pI (25°)
Cytochrome c (horse)	10.6	γ-Globulin (human)	6.6	Lysozyme (hen)	11.0
Fibrinogen (human)	5.5	Histone (bovine)	10.8	Ribonuclease A (bovine)	9.4
Haemoglobin A (human)	7.1	Insulin (human)	5.4	Serum albumin (human)	4.9

1.4 Carbohydrates

Carbohydrates, or sugars as they are commonly known, are classified as monosaccharides, oligosaccharides and polysaccharides. **Monosaccharides** are either polyhydroxyaldehydes (**aldoses**) or polyhydroxyketones (**ketoses**), which are not converted to any simpler polyhydroxyaldehydes and polyhydroxyketones respectively under aqueous hydrolysis conditions. Carbohydrates also include compounds such as glucosamine (Figure 1.10), whose structures contain amino groups as well as hydroxy groups. These compounds are known as **amino sugars**. However, not all polyhydroxyaldehydes and ketones are classified as carbohydrates.

Monosaccharides are classified according to the total number of carbon atoms in their structure. For example, an aldohexose is a monosaccharide that contains a total of six carbon atoms including that of the aldehyde in its structure. Similarly, a ketopentose has five carbons in its structure including the one in the keto group. **Oligosaccharides** are carbohydrates that yield from two to about nine monosaccharide molecules when one molecule of the oligosaccharide is hydrolysed. Small oligosaccharides are often classified according to the number of monosaccharide residues contained in their structures. For example, disaccharides and trisaccharides contain two and three monosaccharide residues respectively whilst **polysaccharides** yield larger numbers of monosaccharide molecules per polysaccharide molecule on hydrolysis. All types of carbohydrate occur widely in the human body. They exhibit a wide variety of biological functions but in particular act as major energy sources for the body.

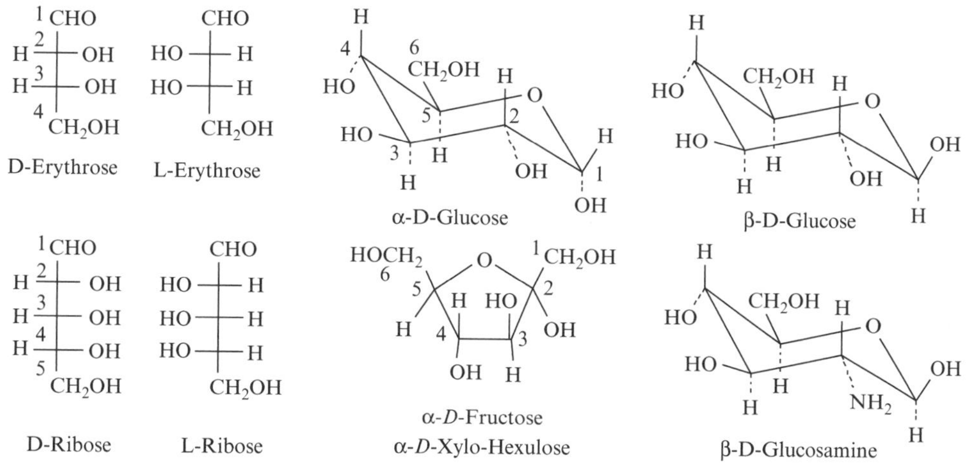

Figure 1.10   Examples of the cyclic and straight chain structures of monosaccharides. The carbon of the carbonyl group has the lowest locant

1.4.1   The structure of monosaccharides

Monosaccharides can exist as either straight chain or cyclic structures (Figure 1.10). Those with five or more carbon atoms usually assume either a five (**furanose**) or six (**pyranose**) membered ring structure. These cyclic structures are formed by an internal nucleophilic addition between a suitably positioned hydroxy group in the molecule and the carbonyl group (Figure 1.11). It results in the formation of the corresponding cyclic hemiacetal or hemiketal. The rings of these cyclic products exist in their normal conformations. For example, six

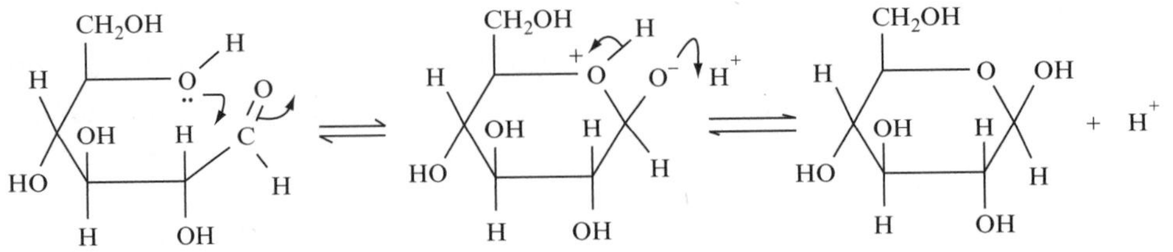

Figure 1.11 The cyclization of the *straight chain* form of glucose to form the β-hemiacetal cyclic form of the molecule

membered rings usually occur as chair conformations whilst five membered rings exist as envelope conformations.

This internal nucleophilic addition introduces a new chiral centre into the molecule. The carbon of the new centre is known as the **anomeric carbon** and the two new stereoisomers formed are referred to as **anomers**. The isomer where the new hydroxy group and the CH_2OH are on opposite sides of the plane of the ring is known as the alpha (α) anomer. Conversely, the isomer with the new hydroxy group and terminal CH_2OH on the same side of the plane of the ring is known as the beta (β) anomer (Figure 1.12).

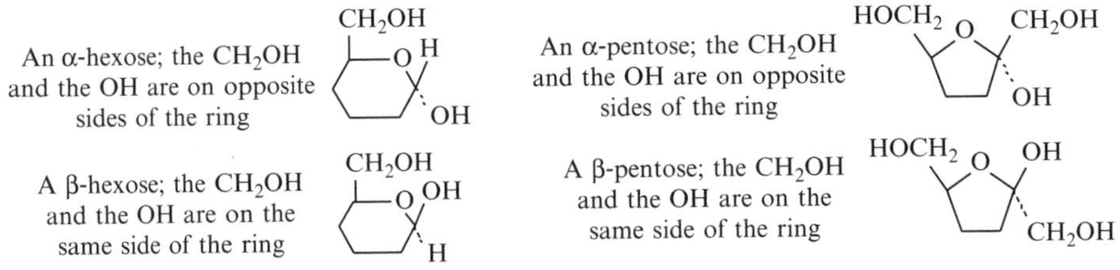

Figure 1.12 The α- and β-anomers of monosaccharides drawn using the Haworth convention. In this convention solid lines represent bonds above the plane of the ring whilst dotted lines are used to indicate bonds below the plane of the ring. Reproduced from G Thomas, *Chemistry for Pharmacy and the Life Sciences including Pharmacology and Biomedical Science*, 1996, by permission of Prentice Hall, a Pearson Education Company

In many cases pure α- and β-anomers may be obtained by using appropriate isolation techniques. For example, crystallization of D-glucose from ethanol yields α-D-glucose $[α]_D$ +112.2° whilst crystallization from aqueous ethanol produces β-D-glucose $[α]_D$ +18.7°. In the solid state these forms are stable and do not interconvert. However, in aqueous solution these cyclic structures can form equilibrium mixtures with the corresponding straight chain form (Figure 1.13). The change in optical rotation due to the conversion of either the pure α- or pure β-anomer of a monosaccharide into an equilibrium mixture of both forms in aqueous solution is known as **mutarotation** (Figure 1.13).

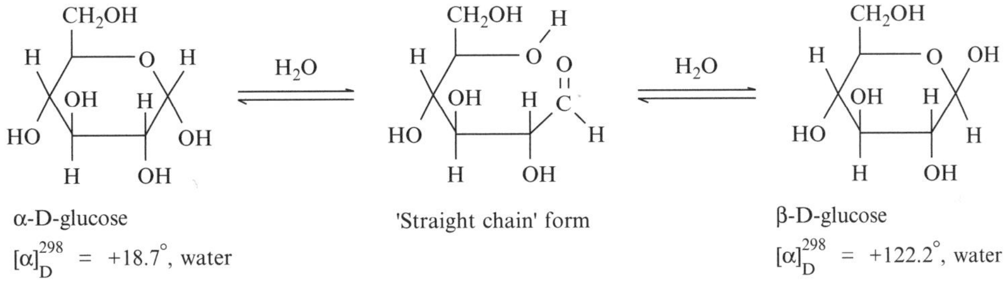

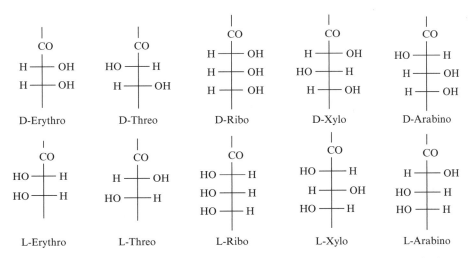

α-D-glucose

$[\alpha]_D^{298} = +18.7°$, water

'Straight chain' form

β-D-glucose

$[\alpha]_D^{298} = +122.2°$, water

Figure 1.13 The mutarotation of glucose anomers. The specific rotation of the aqueous equilibrium mixture is +52°

All monosaccharides have a number of stereogenic centres. The configurations of these centres may be indicated by the use of the R/S nomenclature system. However, the historic system where the configurations of all the chiral centres are indicated by the stem name of the monosaccharide (Figure 1.14) is generally preferred. In addition, monosaccharides are also classified as D or L according to the configuration of their pentultimate CHOH group. In the D form this hydroxy group **projects on the right** of the carbon chain towards the observer whilst in the L form it **projects on the left** of the carbon chain towards the observer when the molecule is viewed with the unsaturated group at the top. These configurations are usually represented, on paper, by modified Fischer projections (Figure 1.14) with the unsaturated group drawn at the top of the chain. The D and L forms of a monosaccharide have mirror image structures, that is, are enantiomers (Figure 1.10).

D-Erythro   D-Threo   D-Ribo   D-Xylo   D-Arabino

L-Erythro   L-Threo   L-Ribo   L-Xylo   L-Arabino

Figure 1.14 Examples of the stem names used to indicate the configurations of the chiral centres in monosaccharides. The system is based on the relative positions of adjacent hydroxy groups with the carbonyl group being used as a reference point for the hydroxy groups. L configurations are mirror images of the corresponding D configurations.

Some monosaccharides may also be classified as being **epimers**. Epimers are compounds that have identical configurations except for one carbon atom. For example, α-D-glucose and α-D-fructose are epimers. Epimers sometimes react with the same reagent to form the same product. For example, both α-D-glucose and α-D-fructose react with phenylhydrazine to form the same osazone.

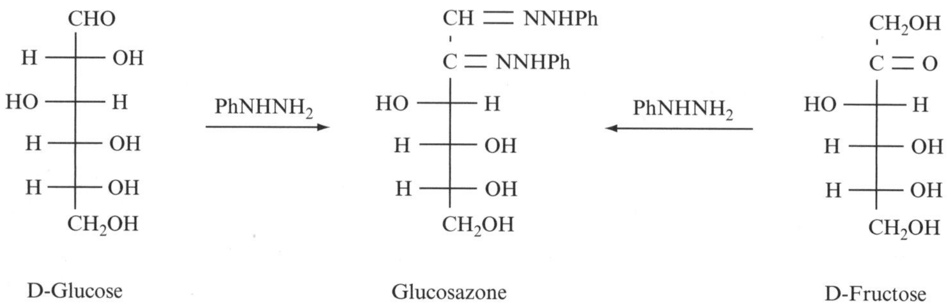

| | CHO | | | CH = NNHPh | | | CH₂OH |
The chemical properties of monosaccharides are further complicated by the fact that they can exhibit tautomerism in aqueous basic solutions (Figure 1.15). This means that after a short time a basic aqueous solution of a monosaccharide will also contain a mixture of monosaccharides that will exhibit their characteristic chemical properties. For example, a solution of fructose will produce a silver mirror when treated with an ammoniacal solution of silver nitrate (Tollen's reagent). This is because under basic conditions fructose undergoes tautomerism to glucose, whose structure contains an aldehyde group, which reduces Tollen's reagent to metallic silver.

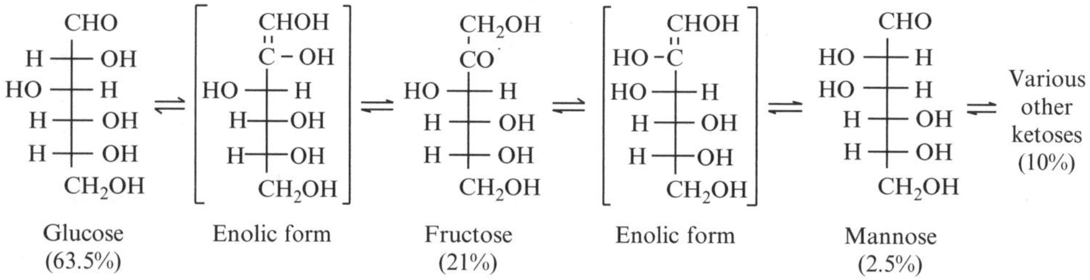

Figure 1.15 The tautomerism of glucose in a basic aqueous solution. The approximate concentrations of the isomers present at equilibrium are given in the brackets

1.4.2 The nomenclature of monosaccharides

Monosaccharides are normally known by their traditional trivial names. However, systematic names are in use. The systematic names of 'straight chain'

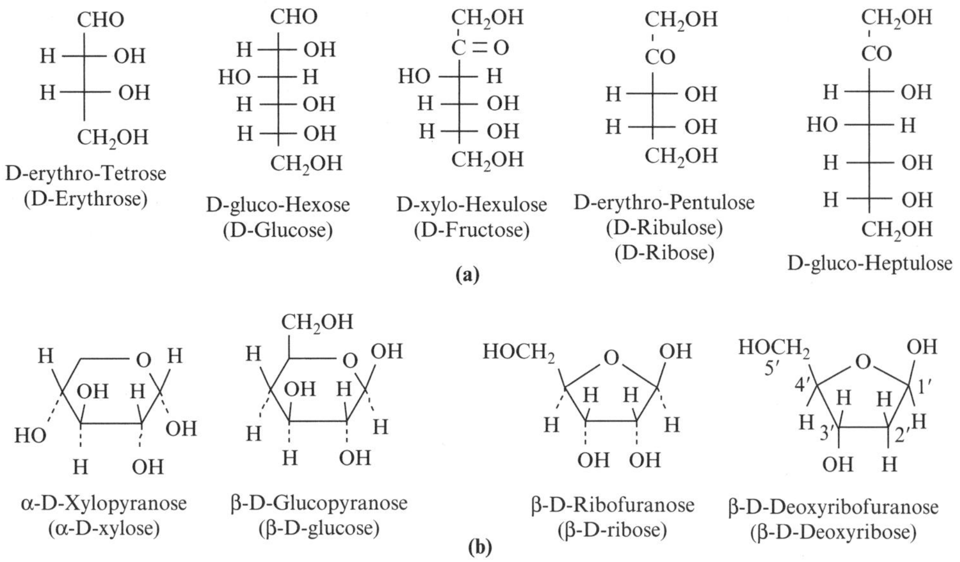

Figure 1.16 Monosaccharide nomenclature. Commonly used trivial names are given in the brackets

monosaccharides are based on a stem name indicating the number of carbon atoms, a prefix indicating the configuration of the hydroxy group and either the suffix **-ose** (aldoses) or **-ulose** (ketoses). In addition the name is also prefixed by the D or L as appropriate (Figure 1.16(a)). Five membered ring monosaccharides have the stem name **furanose** whilst six membered ring compounds have the stem name **pyranose** together with the appropriate configurational prefixes indicating the stereochemistry of the anomers (Figure 1.16(b)). Monosaccharides in which one of the hydroxy groups has been replaced by a hydrogen atom have the prefix **deoxy-** with the appropriate locant, except if it is at position 2, when no locant is given.

1.4.3 Glycosides

Many endogenous compounds occur as **glycosides**. These are compounds which consist of a carbohydrate residue, known generally as a **glycone**, bonded to a non-sugar residue, known generally as an **aglycone**, by a so called **glycosidic link** to the anomeric carbon of the glycone. Since the glycosidic link is formed to the anomeric carbon both α- and β-isomers of a glycoside are known. The structures of glycosidic links vary, the most common being an ether group (oxygen glycosidic links) but amino (nitrogen glycosidic links), sulphide (sulphur glycosidic links) and carbon to carbon links (carbon glycosidic links) are known (Figure 1.17). Each type of glycosidic link will exhibit the characteristics of the structure forming the link. For example, oxygen glycosidic links are effectively acetals and so undergo hydrolysis in aqueous solution. Both trivial and systematic nomenclature is used for glycosides (Figure 1.17). In systematic nomenclature the radical name of the aglycone preceeds the name of the glycone, which has the suffix **-oside**.

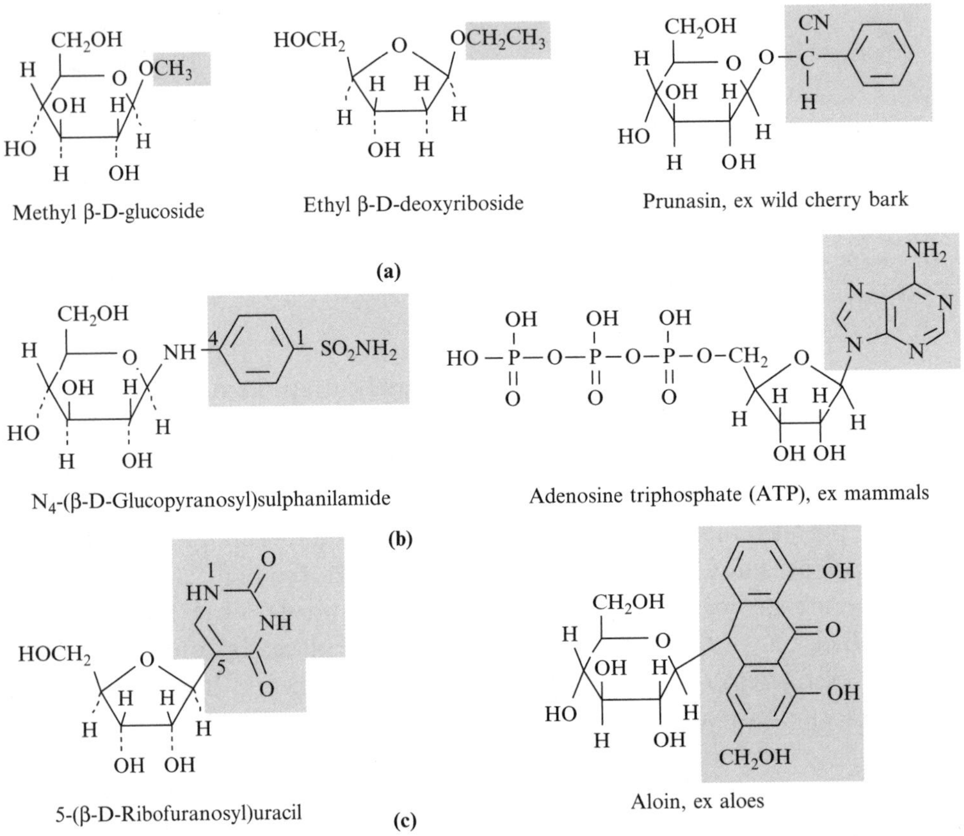

Methyl β-D-glucoside

Ethyl β-D-deoxyriboside

Prunasin, ex wild cherry bark

(a)

N₄-(β-D-Glucopyranosyl)sulphanilamide

Adenosine triphosphate (ATP), ex mammals

(b)

5-(β-D-Ribofuranosyl)uracil

(c)

Aloin, ex aloes

Figure 1.17 Examples of (a) oxygen glycosides, (b) nitrogen glycosides and (c) carbon glycosides. The shaded parts of the structures are the aglycone sections

Glycoproteins are glycosides that have a protein aglycone. The protein is usually linked to a polysacharide (See section 1.4.4) by an O or N glycosidic link. Glycoproteins are found in all forms of life. They exhibit a wide range of biological activities. For example, they may act as receptors, hormones and enzymes.

1.4.4 Polysaccharides

Polysaccharides (**glycans**) are carbohydrates whose structures consist of monosaccharide residues joined together by oxygen glycosidic linkages (Figure 1.18).

The links between between monosaccharide residues of a polysaccharide molecule are usually referred to in terms of the type of the numbers of the carbon atoms forming the link and the stereochemistry of the anomeric position. For example, the glycosidic link formed in maltose is refered to as an α-1,4-link (Figure 1.19) because the anomeric carbon of an α-D-glucose residue is linked to carbon number 4 of the other (second) glucose residue in the structure. The anomeric carbon atom of the second glucose residue can undergo mutarotation and so maltose will exist as two isomers in aqueous solution. The prefix (α, β) is used for residues that can undergo mutarotation.

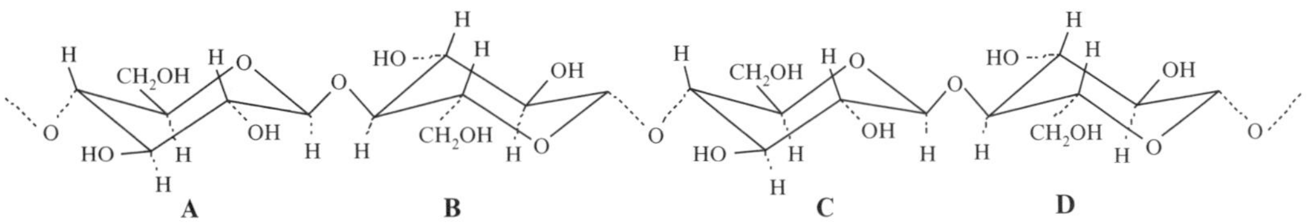

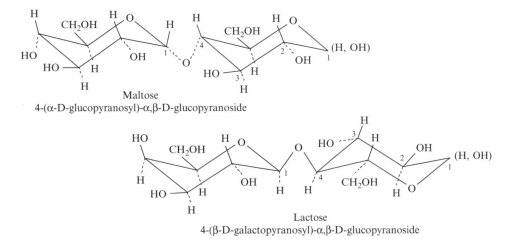

Figure 1.18 A fragment of the β-D-glucose chain in cellulose

Maltose
4-(α-D-glucopyranosyl)-α,β-D-glucopyranoside

Lactose
4-(β-D-galactopyranosyl)-α,β-D-glucopyranoside

Figure 1.19 Examples of simple disaccharides. Appropriate systematic names are given in brackets. The structures are normally drawn so that the oxygen atom forming the glycosidic link is above or below the plane of the ring system. This sometimes requires the structure of a residue to be turned around and/or over in order to obtain the correct alignment of the oxygen atom. Hexagonal cardboard cutouts can be useful in determining how a particular glycosidic link was formed

The stereochemical nature of these oxygen glycosidic links is important in the control of the metabolism of polysaccharides. Enzymes that catalyse the aqueous hydrolysis of the glycosidic links of polysaccharides will only usually catalyse the cleavage of a link formed by a particular anomer or anomers. For example, an α-glucosidase catalyses the hydrolysis of glycosidic links formed by an α-glucose residue acting as a glycone in the polysaccharide chain.

1.4.5   The nomenclature of polysaccharides

Trivial names are normally used for all types of polysaccharide. Systematic names may be used for small polysaccharides. These names are based on the systematic names of the monosaccharides corresponding to the residues. However, the suffix **-osyl** is used for a substituent residue joined through its anomeric carbon to the next residue in the chain and the suffix **-oside** is used for the last residue in the chain (Figure 1.19). Appropriate locants may or may not be used in systematic names.

1.4.6   Naturally occurring polysaccharides

Naturally occurring polysaccharides can occur either as individual carbohydrate molecules or in combination with other naturally occurring substances, such as proteins (glycoproteins) and lipids (glycolipids). In all cases the polysaccharide section may have linear or branched chain structures, which often contain the derivatives of both monosaccharides and aminosugars (Figure 1.20).

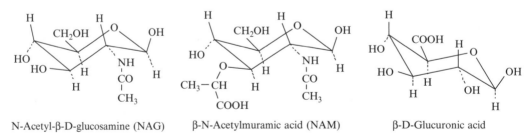

N-Acetyl-β-D-glucosamine (NAG)   β-N-Acetylmuramic acid (NAM)   β-D-Glucuronic acid

Figure 1.20   Some derivatives of monosaccharides and amino sugars commonly found in polysaccharides

Polysaccharides and molecules whose structures contain polysaccharide residues have a wide variety of biochemical roles. They occur as integral parts of the structures of specific tissues: the mureins, for example, (Figure 1.21(a)) are glycoproteins that form part of the cell walls of bacteria (Appendix 3) while the chondroitins are glycosaminoglycans that occur in cartilage, skin and connective tissue. Other polysaccharides have specific biological activities. For example, heparin inhibits the clotting of blood whilst starch and glycogen (Figure 1.21b), are the main energy stores of mammals, plants and microorganisms. Polysaccharide residues also form parts of some enzyme and receptor molecules.

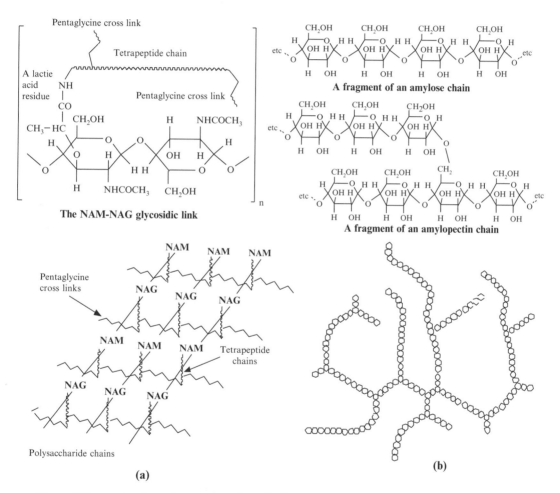

Figure 1.21 (a) A schematic representation of a fragment of the structure of the glycoprotein (a murein) forming the cell wall of Gram-positive bacteria. Adapted from G Thomas *Medicinal Chemistry, an Introduction*, 2000, John Wiley and Sons, Ltd. (b) A representation of the structure of glycogen and starch. Both structures are based on chains of α-glucose residues joined by α-(1,4) glycosidic links in a similar manner to that found in amylose. In glycogen, these chains are branched every eight to 10 glucose residues, the branches being attached by α-(1,6) glycosidic links similar to those found in the amylopectins. Starch consists of unbranched amylose chains (10–20%) and amylopectins with branches occurring every 20–30 glucose residues

1.5   Lipids

1.5.1   Introduction

The term lipid is the collective name given to a wide variety of classes of naturally occurring compounds isolated from plant and animal material by extraction with nonpolar solvents. This section discusses a selection of the classes of compound that are classified as lipids. However, not all classes of compound obtained by extraction with nonpolar solvents are classified as lipids.

1.5.2   Fatty acids

This is the most abundant group of compounds that are classified as lipids. They occur as isolated molecules and are more commonly found as residues in other lipid structures. The fatty acids and residues that are commonly found are normally referred to by trivial names (Table 1.4). They usually have 'straight chain structures' with even numbers of between 14 and 22 carbon atoms inclusive. Both saturated and unsaturated residues are found. In the latter case both *cis* and *trans* isomers are known but the *cis* isomers are more common. A few residues have structures that have side chains and/or other functional groups.

Table 1.4   Fatty acids that are commonly found in lipids. Ricinoleic acid is optically active because its number 12 carbon atom is chiral

Trivial name	Systematic name	Structure
Palmitic acid	Hexadecanoic acid	$CH_3(CH_2)_{14}COOH$
Palmitoleic acid	*cis*-Hexadecenoic acid	$CH_3(CH_2)_5CH = CH(CH_2)_7COOH$
Stearic acid	Octadecanoic acid	$CH_3(CH_2)_{16}COOH$
Oleic acid	*cis*-9-Octadecanoic acid	$CH_3(CH_2)_7CH = CH(CH_2)_7COOH$
Linoleic acid	*cis*-9-*cis*-12-Octadecadienoic acid	$CH_3(CH_2)_3(CH_2CH = CH)_2(CH_2)_7COOH$
Linolenic acid	*cis*-9-*cis*-12-*cis*-15-Octadecatrienoic acid	$CH_3(CH_2CH = CH)_3(CH_2)_7COOH$
Ricinoleic acid	12-hydroxy-*cis*-9-Octadecanoicacid	$CH_3(CH_2)_5CHOHCH_2CH = CH(CH_2)_7COOH$
Arachidonic acid	*cis*-5-*cis*-8-*cis*-11-*cis*-14-Eicosatetraenoic acid	$CH_3(CH_2)_3(CH_2CH = CH)_4(CH_2)_3COOH$

1.5.3 Acylglycerols (glycerides)

Acylglycerols are the mono-, di- and tri-esters of glycerol and fatty acids (Figure 1.22). The fatty acid residues of di- and tri-esters may or may not be the same. Tri-esters are the most common naturally occuring acylglycerols.

Complex mixtures of acylglycerols are the major components of naturally occuring fats and oils. Oils are fats that are liquid at room temperature. Their liquidity is attributed to their acid residues having a high proportion of $C=C$ bonds. Triacylglycerols are the predominant energy store in animals and are mainly located in adipose tissue.

Metabolism of fats is responsible for supplying a significant part of the energy requirements of many cells. Initially the fat is hydrolysed to glycerol and the appropriate fatty acids. Metabolic oxidation of these fatty acids liberates energy in a form that can be utilized by the cell.

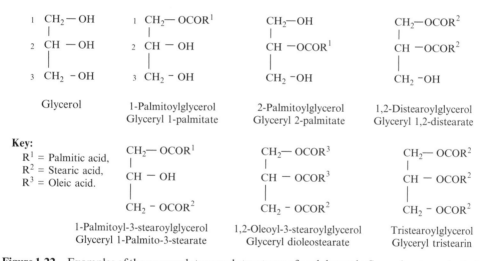

Figure 1.22 Examples of the nomenclature and structures of acylglycerols. Several systems, including the IUPAC system for esters, are used to name acylglycerols. In addition to the IUPAC system, two nomenclature systems are in common use. The first uses glycerol as a stem name, the fatty acid residues being indicated by their acyl prefixes together with an appropriate locant. The second system uses glyceryl followed by the names of the acid residues arranged in the order they appear in the molecule. However, the ending -*ic* of the acid is replaced by the suffix -*o* except for the last residue, which is given the ending -*ate*. The suffix -*in* is used when all three fatty acid residues are identical

1.5.4 Steroids

Steroids are compounds based on fused multi-ring carbon skeletons, each ring being referred to by a letter (Figure 1.23(a)). The rings may be saturated or

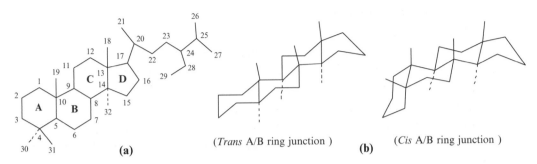

Figure 1.23 (a) The ring and number system of steroids. (b) The conformations of the ring junctions found in steroids with saturated rings

unsaturated and in some compounds ring A is a benzene ring. Six membered saturated rings usually have a chair conformation whilst the five membered saturated rings have an envelope configuration. For steroids with saturated A and B rings with chair conformations the substituents at the A/B ring junction can be *trans* or *cis* but those of the B/C and C/D ring junction are usually *trans* (Figure 1.23(b)). Bonds that lie in the plane or project above the plane of the rings are known as β-bonds (solid lines) whilst bonds that are directed below the plane of the rings are designated as α-bonds (dotted lines). The traditional number system used for steroids is also extended to include their side chains. Many steroids are biologically important. Cholesterol, for example, is an important component of mammalian cell membranes (Appendix 3), whilst ergosterol (Figure 1.24) occurs in the cell membranes of fungi. Steroids such as testosterone and oestradiol act as hormones.

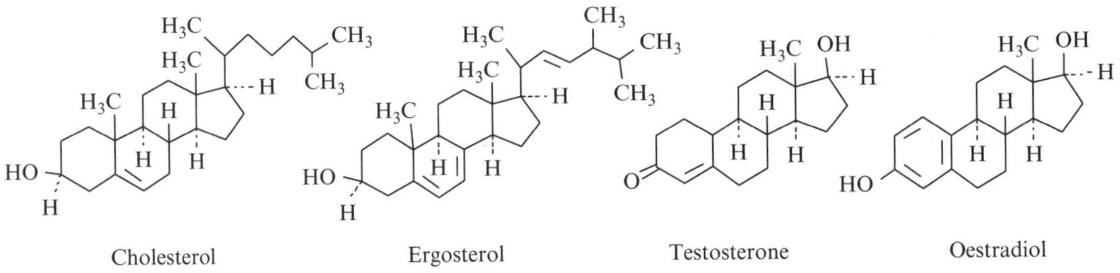

Cholesterol   Ergosterol   Testosterone   Oestradiol

Figure 1.24 Examples of some important naturally occuring steroids

1.5.5 Terpenes

Terpenes are compounds whose carbon skeletons can be artifically divided into isoprene units (Figure 1.25), although there are some exceptions to this rule.

Consequently, their carbon skeletons usually contain five or multiples of five carbon atoms. The structures of terpenes may also contain functional groups, such as alcohols, ethers, esters and ketones.

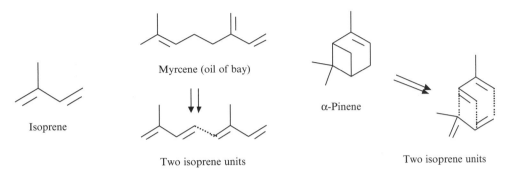

Figure 1.25 The isoprene rule for classifying compounds as terpenes. To apply the rule one ignores the double bonds (see myrcene) and in some cases it is also necessary to distort the isoprene structure (see α-pinene)

Most terpenes are known by their historic trivial names, although systematic names may be used for simple compounds. Terpenes are also classified according to the number of carbon atoms in their structures (Table 1.5).

Table 1.5 The classification system for terpenes

Number of C atoms	Classification
10	Monoterpene
15	Sesquiterpene
20	Diterpene
25	Sesterterpene
30	Triterpene
40	Tetraterpene

Monoterpenes are the main constituents of a group of compounds that are known as the **essential oils**. They are extracted from plants and animals and have been used as perfumes, medicines and spices for thousands of years (Figure 1.26).

1.5.6 Phospholipids

Most phospholipids are essentially disubstituted phosphates (Figure 1.27). They may be initially classified as phosphatidyl compounds, plasmalogens, ether phospholipids and sphingomyelins depending on the nature of the R_1 group attached to the phosphate residue (Table 1.6).

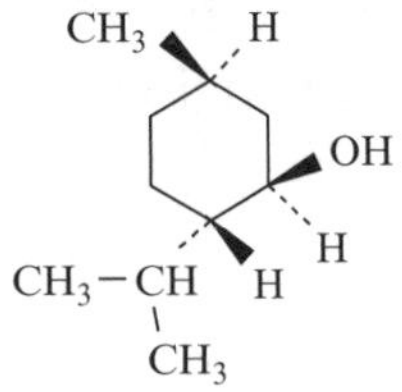

Menthol
(counter-irritant)   Eucalyptol 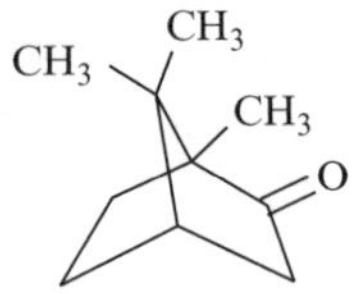   Camphor 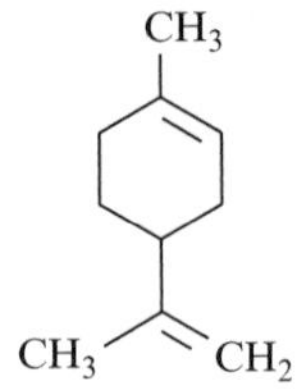   Limonene
                                                                                   (Lemon grass oil)

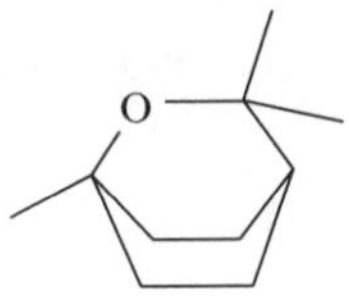

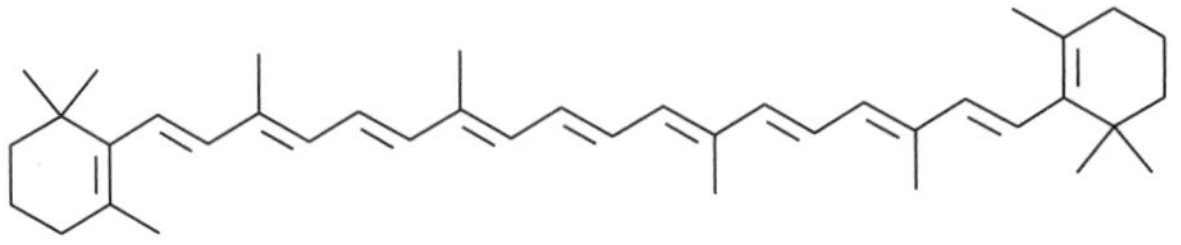

β-Carotene (Precursor of vitamin A and anti-oxidant)

Figure 1.26   Examples of naturally occuring terpenes

Figure 1.27   A disubstituted phosphate

Table 1.6   The classification of phospholipids according to the nature of their R_1 group. R groups have long hydrocarbon chains, the same as those found in fatty acids. The R groups in a particular molecule do not have to have the same structures

Classification	R_1
Phosphatidyl lipids	RCOO — CH$_2$ | RCOO — CH | CH$_2$ —
Ether phospholipids	CH$_2$ – OR | RCOO — CH | CH$_2$ —
Plasmalogens	CH$_2$ - O — CH = CHR | RCOO — CH | CH$_2$ —
Sphingomyelins	OH | CH$_3$(CH$_2$)$_{12}$CH = CHCHCHCH$_2$ —— | RCONH

Table 1.7 Examples of the classification of α-phosphatidyl lipids. Common names are given in brackets

R_2	Classification	Glycerol	Phosphatidyl glycerol
Choline	Phosphatidyl choline (lecithins)	Inositol	Phosphatidyl inositol
Serine	Phosphatidyl serine	Ethanolamine	Phosphatidyl ethanolamine (α-cephalins)

The α-phosphatidyl lipids are further subdivided according to the nature of their R_2 residues (Table 1.7). The R_2 groups of plasmalogens and ether phospholipids are similar to the R_2 groups of the phosphatidyl lipids, whilst the sphingomyelins have a choline residue.

Phospholipid molecules form the lipid bilayer of cell membranes (Appendix 3). Plasmalogens and sphingomyelins are particularly abundant in brain tissue.

1.5.7 Glycolipids

Most glycolipids are glycosides with a sphingosine derivative (ceramide) acting as the aglycone. They are subdivided according to the nature of the carbohydrate residue (Table 1.8).

Cerebrosides occur mainly in brain and nervous tissues. Sulphatides are the main sulpholipids in the brain, where they account for approximately 15% of the white matter. Gangliosides are particularly abundant in the cells of the central nervous system. They are believed to be the receptors (Figure A4.1 and Appendix 5) for toxins, such as cholera and tetanus toxins, and some viruses, such as the influenza virus.

Table 1.8 Examples of the subclassification of glycolipids. R groups are normally long saturated hydrocarbon chains with 21–25 carbon atoms (a C22–C26 fatty acid residue)

Subclassification	Structure
Cerebrosides (neutral glycolipids) have either a glucose or galactose carbohydrate residue.	$CH_3(CH_2)_{12}CH = CHCHCHNHCOR$ with OH; A β-D-glucose residue

(continues overleaf)

Table 1.8 (*continued*)

Subclassification	Structure
Sulphatides (acidic glycolipids) have galactose residue with a sulphate group.	
Gangliosides (acidic glycolipids) have a polysaccharide chain which branches through an ether linkage at the point marked Z. A typical branch residue would be sialic acid, shown bottom right.	

1.6   Nucleic acids

1.6.1   Introduction

The nucleic acids are the compounds that are responsible for the storage and transmission of the genetic information that controls the growth, function and reproduction of all types of cell. They are classified into two general types: the **deoxyribonucleic acids (DNA)**, whose structures contains the sugar residue β-D-deoxyribose, and the **ribonucleic acids (RNA)**, whose structures contain the sugar residue β-D-ribose (Figure 1.16). Both types of nucleic acid consist of long polymer chains (Figure 1.28(a)) based on a repeating unit known as a **nucleotide** (Figure 1.28(b)). Each nucleotide consists of a purine or pyrimidine (Figure 1.28(c)) base bonded to the 1′ carbon atom of a sugar residue by a β-N-glycosidic link (Figure 1.28(d)). These sugar–base units, which are known

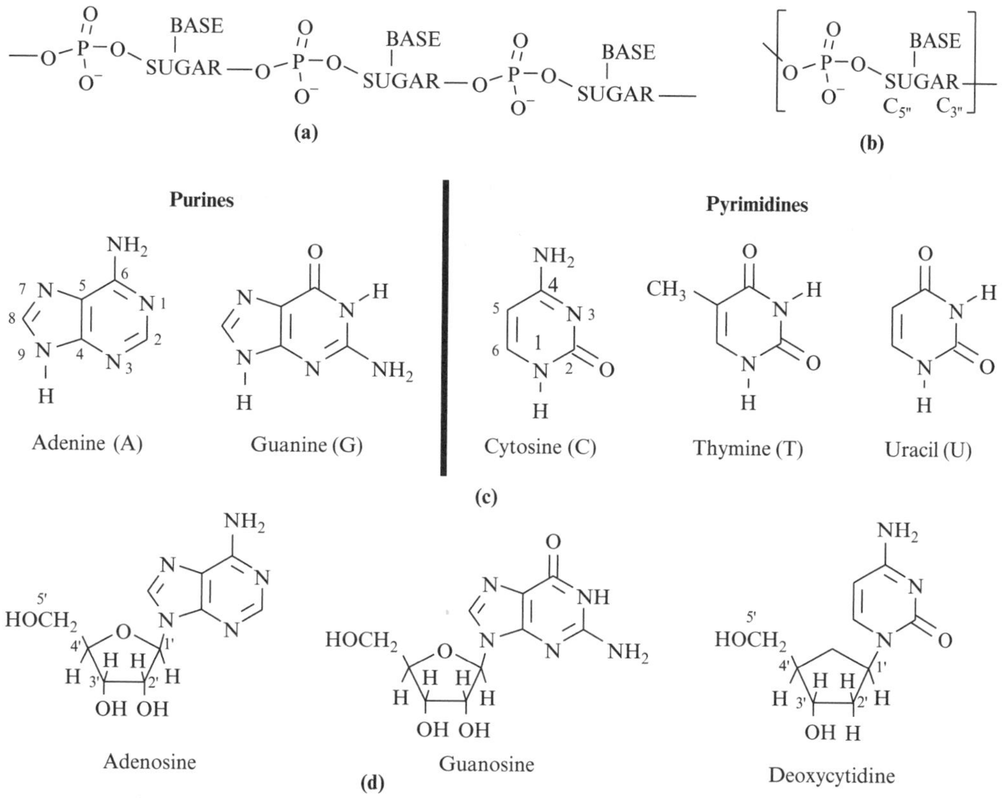

Figure 1.28 (a) The general structure of a nucleotide. (b) A schematic representation of a section of a nucleic acid chain. (c) The bases commonly found in DNA and RNA. These bases are indicated by the appropriate letter in the structures of Nucleic acids. Thymine is not found in RNA; it is replaced by uracil, which is similar in shape and structure. (d) Examples of nucleosides found in DNA and RNA

as **nucleosides** are linked, through the 3′ and 5′ carbons of their sugar residues, by phosphate units to form the nucleic acid polymer chain (Figure 1.28(d)).

Nucleotides can exist as individual molecules with one or more phosphate or polyphosphate groups attached to the sugar residue. The names of these molecules are based on those of the corresponding **nucleosides**. Ribose **nucleosides** are named after their bases (Figure 1.28(c)) but with either the suffix **-osine** or **-idine**. Nucleosides based on deoxyribose use the name of the corresponding RNA nucleoside prefixed by **deoxy-** (Figure 1.28(d)). The purine and pyrimidine rings are numbered in the conventional manner (Figure 1.28(c)) whilst primes are used for the sugar residue numbers (Figure 1.28(d)). Numbers are not included in the name if the phosphate unit is at position 5′ (Figure 1.29). The positions of phosphates attached at any other position are indicated by the appropriate locants.

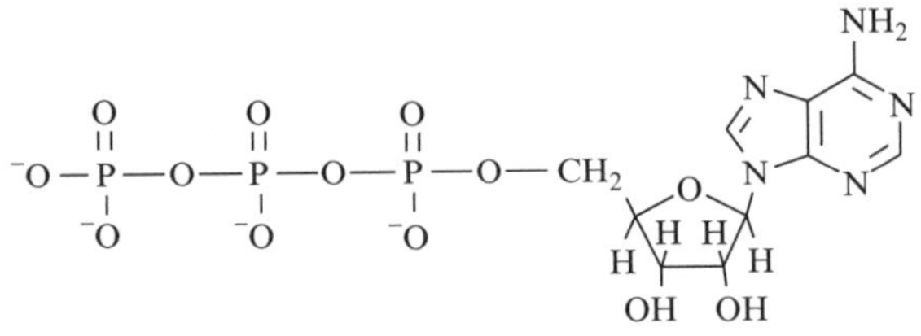

Adenosine triphosphate (ATP)

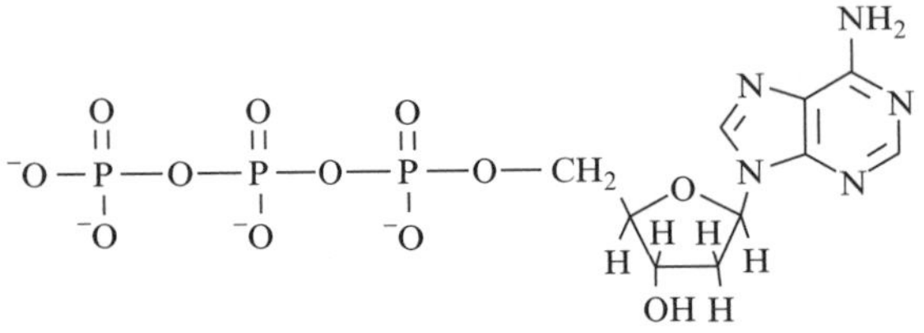

Deoxyadenosine triphosphate (dATP)

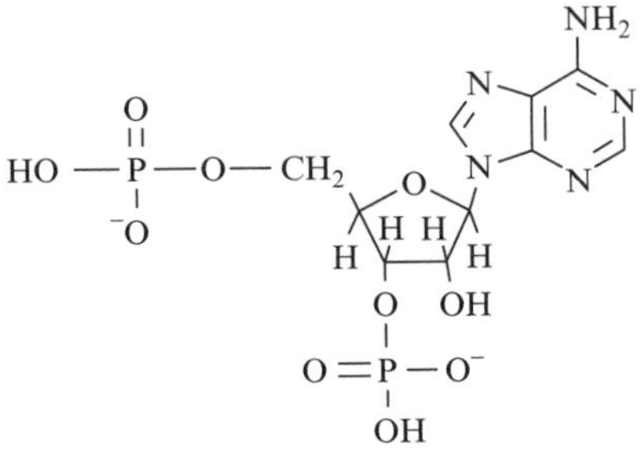

Adenosine 3',5'-diphosphate (3',5'-ADP)

Figure 1.29 Some examples of individual nucleotides. The abbreviations used to represent the structures of nucleotides based on deoxyribose are prefixed by *d* -

1.6.2 DNA, structure and replication

DNA molecules are large, with RMMs up to one trillion (10^{12}). Experimental work by Chargaff and other workers led Crick and Watson to propose that the three dimensional structure of DNA consisted of two single molecule polymer chains held together in the form of a double helix by hydrogen bonding between the same pairs of bases, namely the adenine–thymine and cytosine–guanine base pairs (Figure 1.30). These pairs of bases, which are referred to as **complementary base pairs**, form the internal structure of the helix. They are hydrogen bonded in such a manner that their flat structures lie parallel to one another across the inside of the helix. The two polymer chains forming the helix are aligned in opposite directions. In other words, at the ends of the structure one chain has a free 3'-OH group whilst the other chain has a free 5'-OH group. X-Ray diffraction studies have since confirmed this as the basic three dimensional shape of the polymer chains of the B-DNA, the natural form of DNA. This form of DNA has about 10 bases per turn of the helix. Its outer surface has two grooves, known as the minor and major grooves respectively, which act as the binding sites for many ligands.

Electron microscopy has shown that the double helical chain of DNA is folded, twisted and coiled into quite compact shapes. A number of DNA

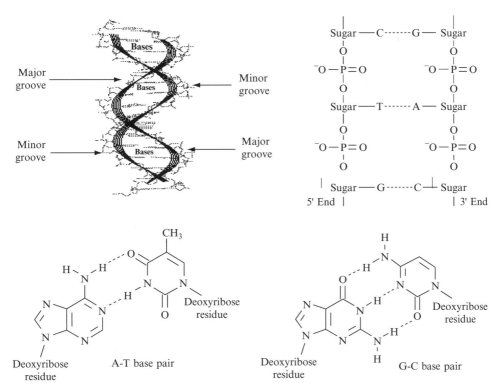

Figure 1.30 The double helical structure of B -DNA. Interchanging of either the bases of a base pair and/or base pair with base pair does not affect the geometry of this structure. Reproduced by permission of Prentice Hall from *Chemistry for Pharmacists and the Life Sciences* by G Thomas

structures are cyclic, and these compounds are also coiled and twisted into specific shapes. These shapes are referred to as supercoils, supertwists and superhelices as appropriate.

DNA molecules are able to reproduce an exact replica of themselves. The process is known as **replication** and occurs when cell division is imminent (Figure 1.31). It is believed to start with the unwinding of the double helix starting at either the end or more usually in a central section, the separated strands acting as templates for the formation of a new **daughter** strand. **New** individual nucleotides bind to these separated strands by hydrogen bonding to the complementary parent nucleotides. As the nucleotides hydrogen bond to the parent strand they are linked to the adjacent nucleotide, which is already hydrogen bonded to the parent strand, by the action of enzymes known as DNA polymerases. As the daughter strands grow the DNA helix continues to unwind. However, **both** daughter strands are formed at the same time in the 5′ to 3′ direction. This means that the growth of the daughter strand that starts at the

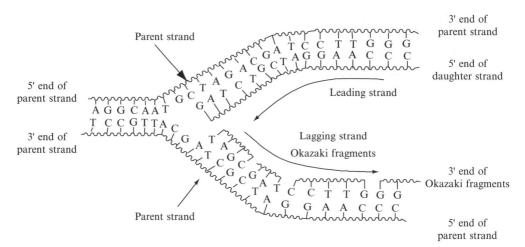

Figure 1.31 A schematic representation of the replication of DNA. The arrows show the directions of the growth of the leading and lagging strands. Hydrogen bonding can only occur between either A and T or C and G. This means that the daughter strand is, in theory, an exact replica of the parent strand. Reproduced by permission of Prentice Hall from *Chemistry for Pharmacists and the Life Sciences* by G Thomas

3′ end of the parent strand can continue smoothly as the DNA helix continues to unwind. This strand is known as the **leading strand**. However, this smooth growth is not possible for the daughter strand that started from the 5′ of the parent strand. This strand, known as the **lagging strand**, is formed in a series of sections, each of which is still grows in the 5′ to 3′ direction. These sections, which are known as Okazaki fragments after their discoverer, are joined together by the enzyme DNA ligase to form the second daughter strand.

Replication, which starts at the end of a DNA helix, continues until the entire structure has been duplicated. The same result is obtained when replication starts at the centre of a DNA helix. In this case unwinding continues in both directions until the complete molecule is duplicated. This latter situation is more common.

1.6.3 Genes and the human genome project

Each species has its own internal and external characteristics, which are determined by the information stored and supplied by the DNA in the nuclei of its cells. The information is carried in the form of a code based on the consecutive sequences of bases found in sections of the DNA structure. This code controls the production of the peptides and proteins required by the body. The sequence of bases that act as the code for the production of one specific peptide or protein molecule is known as a gene.

Genes can normally contain from several hundred to two thousand bases. In simple organisms, such as bacteria, genetic information is usually stored in a continuous sequence of DNA bases. However, in higher organisms the bases forming a particular gene may occur in a number of separate sections known as **exons** separated by sections of DNA that do not appear to be a code for any process. These noncoding sections are referred to as **introns** (Figure 1.32). A number of medical conditions have been attributed to either the absence of a gene or the presence of a degenerate or faulty gene in which one or more of the bases in the sequence have been changed.

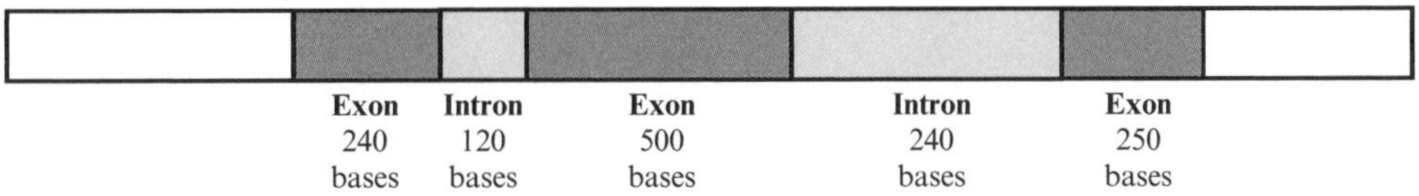

| | Exon
240
bases | Intron
120
bases | Exon
500
bases | Intron
240
bases | Exon
250
bases | |

Figure 1.32 A schematic representation of the gene responsible for the control of the production of the β-subunit of haemoglobin

The complete set of genes that contain all the hereditary information of a particular species is called a **genome**. The Human Genome Project, initiated in 1990, has identified all the genes that occur in humans and also the sequence of bases in these genes.

1.6.4 RNA, structure and transcription

Ribonucleic acids are found in both the nucleus and the cytoplasm. In the cytoplasm RNA is located mainly in small spherical organelles known as **ribosomes**, which consist of about 65% RNA and 35% protein.

The structures of RNA molecules consist of a single polymer chain of nucleotides with the same bases as DNA, with the exception of thymine, which is replaced by uracil, which forms a complementary base pair with adenine (Figure 1.33(a)). These chains often form single stranded **hairpin loops** separated by short sections of a distorted double helix formed by hydrogen bonded complementary base pairs (Figure 1.33(b)).

All types of RNA are formed from DNA by a process known as **transcription**, which occurs in the nucleus. It is thought that the DNA unwinds and the RNA molecule is formed in the 5' to 3' direction. It proceeds smoothly with the 3' end of the new strand bonding to the 5' end of the next nucleotide (Fig. 1.34). This

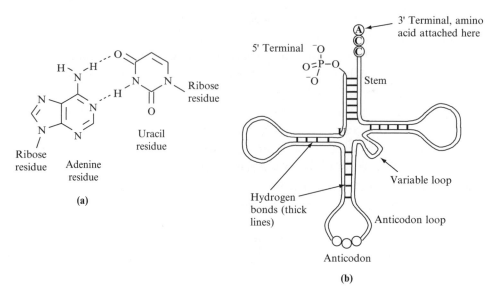

Figure 1.33 (a) The hydrogen bonding between uracil and adenine. (b) The two dimensional cloverleaf representation of the structure of transfer RNA (tRNA) showing the hairpin loops in the structure

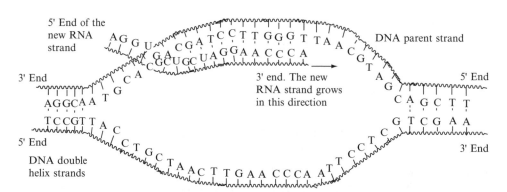

Figure 1.34 A schematic representation of a transcription process. Reproduced from G Thomas, *Chemistry for Pharmacists and the Life Sciences*, 1996, by permission of Prentice-Hall, a Pearson Education Company

bonding is catalysed by enzymes known as RNA polymerases. Since only complementary base pairs can hydrogen bond, the order of bases in the new RNA strand is determined by the sequence of bases in the parent DNA strand. In this way DNA controls the genetic information being transcribed into the RNA molecule. This information is in the form of a series of exons and introns complementary to those found in the parent gene. The strands of DNA contain start and stop signals, which control the size of the RNA molecule produced. These signals are in the form of specific sequences of bases. The RNA produced by transcription is known as either **heterogeneous nuclear RNA (hnRNA)**, **premessenger RNA (pre-mRNA)** or **primary transcript RNA (ptRNA)**.

1.6.5 Classification and function of RNA

Ribonucleic acids are classified according to their general role in protein synthesis.

Messenger RNA (mRNA) is believed to be produced from the hnRNA formed by transcription in the nucleus. The introns are removed and the remaining exons are spliced together to form a continuous sequence of bases that are complementary to the gene's exons. The mRNA now leaves the nucleus via nuclear pores and carries its message to the ribosome in the cytoplasm. It binds to the ribosome, where it dictates the order in which the amino acids are linked to form the structure of the protein This information is carried in the form of a trinucleotide code known as a **codon**. The nature of a codon is indicated by a sequence of letters corresponding to the 5′ to 3′ order of bases in the trinucleotide. Some amino acids have more than one codon. The mRNA's codon code is known as the **genetic code** (Table 1.9) and is used by all living

Table 1.9 The genetic code. The start codon is always AUG. Some codons act as start and stop signals in protein synthesis. Codons are always written left to right, 5′ to 3′

Code	Amino acid	Code	Amino acid	Code	Amino acid	Code	Amino acid
UUU	Phe	CUU	Leu	AUU	Ile	GUU	Val
UUC	Phe	CUC	Leu	AUC	Ile	GUC	Val
UUA	Leu	CUA	Leu	AUA	Ile	GUA	Val
UUG	Leu	CUG	Leu	AUG	Met	GUG	Val
UCU	Ser	CCU	Pro	ACU	Thr	GCU	Ala
UCC	Ser	CCC	Pro	ACC	Thr	GCC	Ala
UCA	Ser	CCA	Pro	ACA	Thr	GCA	Ala
UCG	Ser	CCG	Pro	ACG	Thr	GCG	Ala
UAU	Tyr	CAU	His	AAU	Asn	GAU	Asp
UAC	Tyr	CAC	His	AAC	Asn	GAC	Asp
UAA	Stop	CAA	Gln	AAA	Lys	GAA	Glu
UAG	Stop	CAG	Gln	AAG	Lys	GAG	Glu
UGU	Cys	CGU	Arg	AGU	Ser	GGU	Gly
UGC	Cys	CGC	Arg	AGC	Ser	GGC	Gly
UGA	Stop	CGA	Arg	AGA	Arg	GGA	Gly
UGG	Trp	CGG	Arg	AGG	Arg	GGG	Gly

matter as the code for protein synthesis. mRNA is synthesized as required and, once its message has been delivered, it is eventually decomposed.

Transfer RNA (tRNA) transports the required amino acids from the cell's amino acid pool to the ribosome. Each type of amino acid can only be transported by its own specific tRNA molecule. The tRNA, together with its amino acid residue, binds to the mRNA already bound to the ribosome. It recognizes the point on the mRNA where it has to deliver its amino acid through the use of a consecutive sequence of three bases known as an **anticodon**, which is found on one of the loops of the tRNA (Figure 1.33(b)). This anticodon binds to the complementary codon of the mRNA. Consequently, the amino acids can only be delivered to specific points on the mRNA, which controls the order in which amino acid residues are added to the growing protein. This growth occurs from the N-terminal end of the protein.

Ribosomal RNA (rRNA) is involved in the protein synthesis. It is found in the ribosomes which occur in the cytoplasm. Ribosomes contain about 35% protein and 65% rRNA. Experimental evidence suggests that rRNA molecules have structures that consist of a single strand of nucleotides whose sequence varies considerably from species to species. The strand is folded and twisted to form a series of single stranded loops separated by sections of double helix, which is believed to be formed by hydrogen bonding between complementary base pairs. The general pattern of loops and helixes is very similar between species even though the sequences of nucleotides are different. However, little is known about the three dimensional structures of rRNA molecules and their interactions with the proteins found in the ribosome.

1.7 Questions

(1) Draw the general structural formula of each of the following classes of compound: (a) a β-amino acid, (b) a nucleotide, (c) a plasmalogen, (d) an α-amino acid, (e) a tripeptide and (f) a diacylglycerol (diglyceride).

(2) Describe, using a suitable example, each of the following: (a) a prosthetic group, (b) a peptide link, (c) a S–S bridge and (d) the tertiary structure of a protein.

(3) Define, by reference to glucose, the meaning of each of the following terms: (a) a monosaccharide, (b) mutarotation, (c) a pyranose ring system, (d) anomers and (e) α- and β-glucosides.

(*continued*)

(4)   List five **general classes** of compound that are collectively known as lipids. Describe the essential differences between (a) plasmalogens and sphingomyelins and (b) cerebrosides, sulphatides and gangliosides.

(5)   Draw, number and letter the saturated ring system found in many steroids. Describe the most common conformations of the rings found in saturated steroid ring systems.

(6)   Distinguish carefully between the members of the following pairs of terms: (a) nucleotide and nucleoside; (b) introns and extrons; (c) codons and anticodons.

(7)   The sequence AATCCGTAGC appears on a DNA strand. What would be the the sequence on (a) the complementary chain of this DNA and (b) a transcribed RNA chain?

(8)   (a) How does RNA differ from DNA? (b) Outline the functions of the three principal types of RNA.

(9)   What is the sequence of amino acid residues in the peptide formed from the mRNA

UUCGUUACUUAGUAGCCCAGUGGUGGGU
ACUAAUGGCUCGAG?

Indicate which end of the peptide is the N-terminus.

2 An Introduction to Drugs and Their Action

2.1 Introduction

The primary objective of medicinal chemistry is the design and discovery of new compounds that are suitable for use as drugs. The discovery of a new drug requires not only its design and synthesis but also the development of testing methods and procedures, which are needed to establish how a substance operates in the body and its suitability for use as a drug. Drug discovery may also require fundamental research into the biological and chemical nature of the diseased state. This and other aspects of drug design and discovery require input from specialists in other fields, such as biology, biochemistry, pharmacology, mathematics, computing and medicine amongst others, and the medicinal chemist to have an outline knowledge of these fields.

This chapter seeks to give a broad overview of medicinal chemistry. It attempts to provide a framework for the topics discussed in greater depth in the succeeding chapters. In addition, it includes some topics of general interest to medicinal chemists.

2.2 What are drugs and why do we need new ones?

Drugs are strictly defined as chemical substances that are used to prevent or cure diseases in humans, animals and plants. The **activity** of a drug is its pharmacological effect on the subject, for example, its analgesic or β-blocker action. Drugs act by interfering with biological processes, so no drug is completely

Fundamentals of Medicinal Chemistry, Edited by Gareth Thomas
© 2003 John Wiley & Sons, Ltd
ISBN 0 470 84306 3 (Hbk), ISBN 0 470 84307 1 (pbk)

safe. All drugs can act as poisons if taken in excess. For example, overdoses of paracetamol can cause coma and death. Furthermore, in addition to their beneficial effects, most drugs have non-beneficial biological effects. Aspirin, which is commonly used to alleviate headaches, may also cause gastric irritation and bleeding. The non-beneficial effects of some drugs, such as cocaine and heroin, are so undesirable that the use of these drugs has to be strictly controlled by legislation. These unwanted effects are commonly referred to as **side effects**.

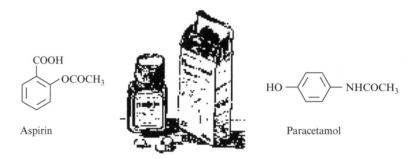

The over-usage of the same drugs, such as antibiotics, can result in the development of resistance to that drug by both the patients, microorganisms and virus the drug is intended to control. Resistance occurs when a drug is no longer effective in controlling a medical condition. Drug resistance or tolerance, often referred to as **tachyphylaxis**, arises in people for a variety of reasons. For example, the effectiveness of barbiturates often decreases with repeated use because repeated dosing causes the body to increase its production in the liver of mixed function oxidases that metabolize the drug, thereby reducing the drug's effectiveness. An increase in the rate of production of an enzyme that metabolizes the drug is a relatively common reason for drug resistance. Another general reason for drug resistance is the **down-regulation** of receptors (Appendix 5). Down-regulation occurs when repeated stimulation of a receptor results in the receptor being broken down. This results in the drug being less effective because there are fewer receptors available for it to act on. Drug resistance may also be due to the appearance of a significantly high proportion of drug resistant strains of microorganisms. These strains arise naturally and can rapidly multiply and become the currently predominant strain of that microorganism. For example, antimalarial drugs are proving less effective because of an increase in the proportion of drug resistant strains of the malaria parasite.

New drugs are constantly required to combat drug resistance, even though it can be minimized by the correct use of medicines by patients. They are also required for the improvement in the treatment of existing diseases, the treatment of newly identified diseases and the production of safer drugs by the reduction or removal of adverse side effects.

2.3 Drug discovery and design, a historical outline

Since ancient times the peoples of the world have used a wide range of natural products for medicinal purposes. These products, obtained from animal, vegetable and mineral sources, were sometimes very effective. However, many of the products were very toxic. Information about these ancient remedies was not readily available to users until the invention of the printing press in the 15th century. This invention led to the widespread publication and circulation of herbals and pharmacopoeias. This resulted in a rapid increase in the use, and misuse, of herbal and other remedies. However, improved communications between practitioners in the 18th and 19th centuries resulted in the progressive removal of preparations that were either ineffective or too toxic from herbals and pharmacopoeias. It also led to a more rational development of new drugs. Initially this development was centred around the natural products isolated from plant and animal material, but as knowledge increased a wider range of pharmaceutically active compounds were used as the starting point for the development of drugs. The compounds on which a development is based are now known as **lead compounds**, while the synthetic compounds developed from a lead are referred to as its **analogues**.

The work of the medicinal chemist is centred around the discovery of new lead compounds with specific medical properties. It includes the development of more effective and safer analogues from both these new and existing lead compounds. This usually involves synthesizing and testing many hundreds of compounds before a suitable compound is produced. It is currently estimated that for every 10 000 compounds synthesized one is suitable for medical use.

The first rational development of synthetic drugs was carried out by Paul Ehrlich and Sacachiro Hata, who produced the antiprotozoal arsphemamine in 1910 by combining synthesis with reliable biological screening and evaluation procedures. Ehrlich, at the begining of the 20th century, had recognized that both the beneficial and toxic properties of a drug were important to its evaluation. He realized that the more effective drugs showed a greater selectivity for the target microorganism than its host. Consequently, to compare the effectiveness of different compounds, he expressed a drug's selectivity, and hence its effectiveness, in terms of its chemotherapeutic index, which he defined as

$$\text{chemotherapeutic index} = \frac{\text{minimum curative dose}}{\text{maximum tolerated dose}} \qquad (2.1)$$

Determination and cataloging of the chemotherapeutic index of the 600 compounds Ehrlich and Hata synthesized enabled them in 1909 to discover arsphemamine (Salvarsan). This drug was very toxic but safer than the then currently used *Atoxyl*. It was used up to the mid-1940s, when it was replaced by penicillin.

Atoxyl   Arsphenamine (Salvarsan)

Today, Ehrlich's chemotherapeutic index has been updated to take into account the variability of individuals and is now defined as its reciprocal, the therapeutic index or ratio:

$$\text{therapeutic index} = \frac{\substack{\text{lethal dose required to kill 50\%} \\ \text{of the test animals (LD}_{50})}}{\substack{\text{the dose producing an effective therapeutic} \\ \text{response in 50\% of the test sample (ED}_{50})}} \qquad (2.2)$$

In theory, the larger a drug's therapeutic index, the greater is its margin of safety. However, in practice index values can only be used as a limited guide to the relative usefulness of different compounds. The term **structure–activity relationship (SAR)** is now used to describe Ehrlich's approach to drug discovery, which consisted of synthesizing and testing a series of structurally related compounds (see section 4.1).

Attempts to quantitatively relate chemical structure to biological action were first initiated in the 19th century, but it was not until the 1960s that Hansch and Fujita devised a method that successfully incorporated quantitative measurements into SAR determinations (see section 4.4). The technique is referred to as **QSAR (quantitative structure–activity relationships)**. One of its most successful uses has been in the development in the 1970s of the antiulcer agents cimetidine and ranitidine. Both SARs and QSARs are important parts of the foundations of medicinal chemistry.

Cimetidine   Ranitidine

An alternative approach to drug design was initiated by the work of John Langley. In 1905 he proposed that so called **receptive substances** in the body could accept either a stimulating compound, which would cause a biological response, or a non-stimulating compound, which would prevent a bio- logical response. It is now universally accepted that the binding of a chemical agent, referred to as a **ligand** (see also section 7.4), to a so called **receptor** sets in motion a series of biochemical events that result in a biological or pharmacological effect. Furthermore, a drug is most effective when its structure or a significant part of its structure, both as regards molecular shape and electron distribution (**stereo- electronic structure**), is complementary with the stereoelectronic structure of the receptor responsible for the desired biological action. The section of the structure of a ligand that binds to a receptor is known as its **pharmacophore**. Furthermore, it is now believed that side effects can arise when the drug binds to either the receptor responsible for the desired biological response or to different receptors.

The mid- to late 20th century has seen an explosion of our understanding of the chemistry of disease states, biological structures and processes. This increase in knowledge has given medicinal chemists a clearer picture of how drugs are distributed through the body and transported across membranes and their mode of operation and metabolism. It has enabled medicinal chemists to place groups that influence absorption, stability in a bio-system, distribution, metabol- ism and excretion in the molecular structure of a drug. For example, the intro- duction of a sulphonic acid group into the structure of a drug will increase its water solubility. This **may** improve its absorption and/or its rate of excretion from the body. However, because of the complex nature of biological systems, there is always a degree of uncertainty in predicting the effect of structural changes on the activity of a drug. As a result, it is always necessary to carry out extensive testing to determine the consequences of modifying a structure. Furthermore, changing a group or introducing a group **may** change the nature of the activity of the compound. For example, the change of the ester group in procaine to an amide (procainamide) changes the activity from a local anaesthetic to anti-rhythmic.

Procaine   Procainamide

The introduction or removal of charged groups or groups that can form ions into or out of a structure may also have a marked affect on drug action. This is because drugs normally have to cross **nonpolar lipid membrane barriers** (Appendix 3) in order to reach their site of action. Consequently, as the polar nature of the drug increases, it usually becomes more difficult for that drug to cross these barriers. For example, quaternary ammonium salts, which are permanently charged, can be used as an alternative to an amine in a structure in order to restrict the passage of a drug across a membrane. The structure of the anticholinesterase neostigmine, developed from physostigmine, contains a quaternary ammonium group, which stops the molecule from crossing the **blood–brain barrier** (Appendix 11). This prevents unwanted CNS activity. However, its analogue miotine can form the free base. As a result, it is able to cross lipid membranes, which may cause unwanted CNS side effects.

Physostigmine

Neostigmine

Miotine

Both SAR and QSAR studies rely on the development team picking the correct starting point. Serendipity inevitably plays a significant part in selecting that point. However, modern techniques such as computer modelling (Chapter 5) and combinatorial chemistry (Chapter 6) introduced in the 1970s and 1990s respectively are likely to reduce the number of intuitive discoveries.

Computer modelling has reduced the need to synthesize every analogue of a lead compound. It is also often used retrospectively to confirm the information derived from other sources. Combinatorial chemistry, which originated in the field of peptide chemistry, has now been expanded to cover other areas. The term covers a group of related techniques for the simultaneous production of large numbers of compounds for biological testing. Consequently, it is used for structure action studies and to discover new lead compounds. The procedures may be automated.

2.4 Sources of drugs and lead compounds

The discovery of a new drug is part luck and part structured investigation (see section 3.1). It originally started with drugs and lead compounds derived from natural sources, such as animals, plants, trees and microorganisms. Marine sources were not utilized to any extent until the mid-20th century. Today, natural sources are still important, but the majority of lead compounds are synthesized in the laboratory. The nature of these synthetic compounds is initially decided from a consideration of the biochemistry of the pathogenic condition.

Today, many discoveries start with biological testing (**bioassays** or **screening programme**) by pharmacologists of the potential sources in order to determine the nature of their pharmacological activity as well as their potencies. These screening programmes may be random or focused. In random screening programs all the substances and compounds available are tested regardless of their structures. The random screening of soil samples, for example, led to the discovery of the streptomycin and tetracycline antibiotics as well as many other lead compounds. Random screening is still employed, but the use of more focused screening procedures where specific structural types are tested is now more common.

Once a screening programme has identified substances of pharmacological activity of interest, the compound responsible for this activity is isolated and used as a lead compound for the production of related analogues. These compounds are subjected to further screening tests. Analogues are made of the most promising of these compounds and they in turn are subjected to the screening procedure. This sequence of selective screening and synthesis of analogues may be repeated many times before a potentially useful drug is found. Often the sequence has to be abandoned as being either unproductive or too expensive.

2.4.1 Natural sources

Natural sources are still important sources of lead compounds and new drugs. However, the large diversity of potential natural sources in the world makes the technique of random screening a rather hit or miss process. The screening of local folk remedies (**ethnopharmacology**) offers the basis of a more systematic approach. In the past this has led to the discovery of many important therapeutic agents, for example, the antimalarial quinine from cinchona bark, the

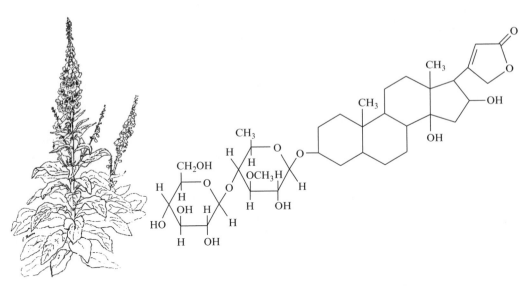

Figure 2.1   The common foxglove and the structure of digitalis

cardiac stimulant digitalis from fox gloves (Figure 2.1) and the antidepressant
reserpine isolated from *Rauwolfia serpentina*.

Once screening identifies a material containing an active compound, the
problem becomes one of extraction, purification and assessment of the pharmacological activity. However, the isolation of useful quantities of a drug from its
land or sea sources can cause ecological problems. The promising anticancer
agent Taxol (Figure 2.2), for example, was originally isolated from the bark
of the Pacific yew tree. However, the production of large quantities of Taxol
from this source would result in the wholesale distruction of the tree, a state
of affairs that is ecologically unacceptable. It is vitally important that plant,
shrub, tree and marine sources of the world are protected from further erosion,

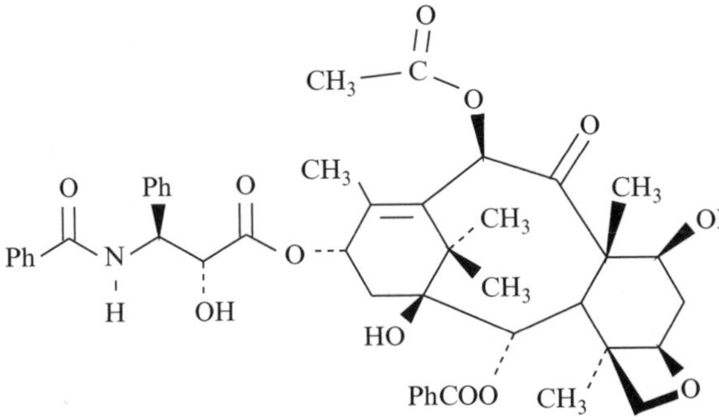

Figure 2.2   Taxol, isolated from the bark of the Pacific yew

as there is no doubt that they will yield further useful therapeutic agents in the future.

2.4.2   Drug synthesis

The most popular approach to drug design by synthesis is to start with the pathology of the diseased state and determine the point where intervention is most likely to be effective (see Chapter 7). This enables the medicinal chemist to suggest possible lead compounds. These compounds are synthesized so that their pharmacological action may be evaluated. Once a suitably active lead is found, structural analogues of that lead are produced and screened in the hope that this procedure will eventually produce a compound that is suitable for clinical use. Obviously this approach is labour intensive and a successful outcome depends a great deal on luck. Various modifications to this approach have been introduced to reduce this element of luck (see Chapters 4–6).

2.4.3   Market forces and 'me-too drugs'

The cost of introducing a new drug to the market is extremely high and continues to escalate. One has to be very sure that a new drug is going to be profitable before it is placed on the market. Consequently, the board of directors' decision to market a drug or not depends largely on information supplied by the accountancy department rather than ethical and medical considerations. One way of cutting costs is for companies to produce drugs with similar activities and molecular structures to their competitors. These drugs are known as the 'me-too drugs'. They serve a useful purpose in that they give the practitioner a choice of medication with similar modes of action. This choice is useful in a number of situations, for example when a patient suffers an adverse reaction to a prescribed drug or on the rare occasion that a drug is withdrawn from the market.

2.5   Classification of drugs

Drugs are classified in a number of different ways depending on where and how the drugs are being used. The methods of most interest to medicinal chemists are chemical structure and pharmacological action, which includes the site of action and target system. Unfortunately, classifying drugs according to their chemical structural type has the disadvantage that members of the same structural group often exhibit very different types of pharmacological activity. Steroids (see section 1.5.4), for example, may act as hormones (testosterone), diuretics (spironolactone) actibacterial agents (fusidic acid) amongst other forms of activity.

The term prodrug (see section 2.7.1 and 9.8) is often used for drugs whose active form is produced by enzyme or chemical action at or near to its site of action. However, it is emphasized that other classifications, such as the nature of the illness and the body system on which the drug acts (physiological classification),

Testosterone   Spironolactone   Fusidic acid

are also used in medicinal chemistry as well as other fields depending on the purpose of the information.

2.6   Routes of administration, the pharmaceutical phase

The physical form in which a medicine is administered is known as its **dosage form**. Dosage forms normally consist of the active constituent and other ingredients known as **excipients**. Excipients can have a number of functions, such as fillers (bulk providing agent), lubricants, binders, preservatives and antioxidants. A change in the nature of the excipients can significantly affect the the stability of the active ingredient as well as its release from the dosage form. Similarly, changes in the preparation of the active principle, such as the use of a different solvent for purification, can affect its bioavailability (see Section 2.7.2 and 8.5) and consequently its effectiveness as a drug. This indicates the importance of quality control procedure for all drugs especially when they reach the manufacturing stage.

The design of dosage forms lies in the field of the pharmaceutical technologist but it should also be considered by the medicinal chemist when developing a

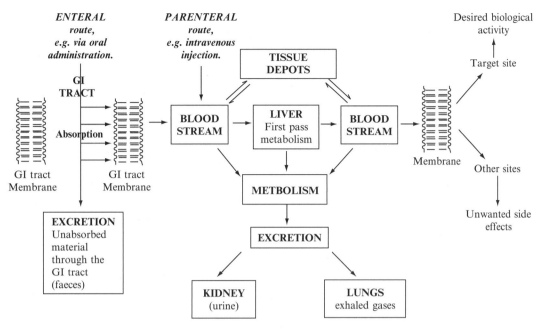

Figure 2.3   The main routes of drug administration and distribution in the body. The distribution of a drug is also modified by metabolism, which can occur at any point in the system

drug from a lead compound. It is no use having a wonder drug if it cannot be packaged in a form that makes it biologically available as well as acceptable to the patient.

Drugs are usually administered topically or systemically. The routes are classified as being either **parenteral** or **enteral** (Figure 2.3). Parenteral routes are those that avoid the gastrointestinal tract (GI. tract), the most usual method being intramuscular injection (IM). The enteral route is where drugs are absorbed from the alimentary canal (PO per oral), rectal and sub-lingual routes. The route selected for the administration of a drug will depend on the chemical stability of the drug, both when it is transported across a membrane (**absorption**) and in transit to the site of action (**distribution**). It will also be influenced by the age, and physical and mental abilities, of the patients using that drug. For example, age related metabolic changes often result in elderly patients requiring lower dosages of the drug to achieve the desired clinical result. Schizophrenics and patients with conditions that require constant medication are particularly at risk of either overdosing or underdosing. In these cases, a slow release intra-muscular injection, which need only be given once in every two to four weeks, rather than a daily dose, may be the most effective use of the medicine.

Consequently, at an appropriately early stage in its development, the design of a drug should also take into account the nature of its target groups.

Once the drug enters the bloodstream it is distributed around the body and, so, a proportion of the drug is either lost by excretion metabolism to other products or is bound to biological sites other than its target site. As a result, the dose administered is inevitably higher than that which would be needed if all the drug reached the appropriate site of biological action. The dose of a drug administered to a patient is the amount that is required to reach and maintain the concentration necessary to produce a favourable response at the site of biological action. Too high a dose usually causes unacceptable side effects whilst too low a dose results in a failure of the therapy. The limits between which the drug is an effective therapeutic agent is known as its **therapeutic window** (Figure 2.4.). The amount of a drug the plasma can contain coupled with processes that irreversibly eliminate (see Section 2.7.14) the drug from its site of action results in the drug concentration reaching a so called **plateau** value. Too high a dose will give a plateau above the therapeutic window and toxic side effects. Too low a dose will result in the plateau below the therapeutic window and ineffective treatment.

The dose of a drug and how it is administered is called the **dosage regimen**. Dosage regimens may vary from a single dose taken to relieve a headache through regular daily doses taken to counteract the effects of epilepsy and diabetes to continuous intravenous infusions for seriously ill patients. Regimens are designed to maintain the concentration of the drug within the therapeutic window at the site of action for the period of time that is required for therapeutic success. The design of the regimen depends on the nature of the medical condition and the medicant. The latter requires not just a knowledge of a drug's biological effects but also its **pharmacokinetic** properties, that is, the rate of its absorption, distribution, metabolism and eliminination from the body.

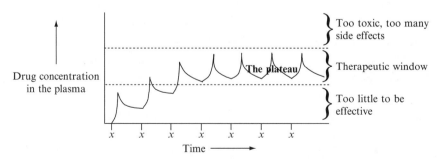

Figure 2.4   A simulation of the therapeutic window for a drug given in fixed doses at fixed time intervals X

2.7   Introduction to drug action

The action of a drug is believed to be due to the interaction of that drug with endogenous and exogenous substrate molecules found in the body (see Chapter 7). When one or more active drug molecules bind to the target endogenous and exogenous molecules, they cause a change or inhibit the biological activity of these molecules. The effectiveness of a drug in bringing about these changes normally depends on the stability of the drug–substrate complex, whereas the medical success of the drug intervention usually depends on whether enough drug molecules bind to sufficient substrate molecules to have a marked effect on the course of the disease state.

The degree of drug activity is directly related to the concentration of the drug in the aqueous medium in contact with the substrate molecules. The factors affecting this concentration in a biological system can be classified into the **pharmacokinetic phase** and the **pharmacodynamic phase** of drug action. The pharmacokinetic phase concerns the study of the parameters that control the journey of the drug from its point of administration to its point of action. The pharmacodynamic phase concerns the chemical nature of the relationship between the drug and its target: in other words, the effect of the drug on the body.

2.7.1   The pharmacokinetic phase

The pharmacokinetic phase of drug action includes the Absorption, Distribution, Metabolism and Elimination (ADME) of the drug. Many of the factors that influence drug action apply to all aspects of the pharmacokinetic phase. Solubility (see Section 3.3), for example, is an important factor in the absorption, distribution and elimination of a drug. Furthermore, the rate of drug dissolution, that is, the rate at which a solid drug dissolves in the aqueous medium, controls its activity when a solid drug is administered by enteral routes (see Section 2.6) as a solid or suspension.

2.7.1.1   Absorption

Absorption is the passage of the drug from its site of administration into the plasma after enteral administration. It involves the passage of the drug through the appropriate membranes. Good absorption normally requires that a drug molecule has the correct balance between its polar (hydrophilic) and nonpolar (hydrophobic) groups. Drugs that are too polar will tend to remain in the bloodstream, whilst those that are too nonpolar will tend to be absorbed into and remain within the lipid interior of the membranes (see Appendix 3). In both cases, depending on the target, the drug is likely to be ineffective.

The degree of absorption can be related to such parameters as partition coefficient, solubility, pK_a, excipients and particle size. For example, the ionization of the analgesic aspirin is suppressed in the stomach by the acids produced from the parietal cells in the stomach lining. As a result, it is absorbed into the bloodstream in significant quantities in its unionized and hence uncharged form through the stomach membrane.

2.7.1.2 Distribution

Distribution is the transport of the drug from its initial point of administration or absorption to its site of action. The main route is the circulatory system; however, some distribution does occur via the lymphatic system. In the former case, once the drug is absorbed, it is rapidly distributed throughout all the areas of the body reached by the blood.

Drugs are transported dissolved in the aqueous medium of the blood either in a 'free form' or reversibly bound to the plasma proteins.

$$\text{Drug} \rightleftharpoons \text{Drug} - \text{Protein complex}$$

Drug molecules bound to plasma proteins have no pharmacological effect until they are released from those proteins. However, it is possible for one drug to displace another from a protein if it forms a more stable complex with that protein. This may result in unwanted side effects, which could cause complications when designing drug regimens involving more than one drug. Moreover, low plasma protein concentrations can affect the distribution of a drug in some diseases, such as rheumatoid arthritis.

Major factors that influence distribution are the solubility (see Section 3.3) and stability (see Biological half life, Section 8.4.1) of drugs in the biological environment of the blood. Sparingly water soluble compounds may be deposited in the blood vessels, leading to restriction in blood flow. Drug stability is of particular importance in that serum proteins can act as enzymes that catalyse the breakdown of the drug. Decompositions such as these can result in a higher dose of the drug being needed in order to achieve the desired pharmacological effect, which increases the risk oftoxic side effects in the patient. However, the active form of some drugs is produced by the decomposition of the administered drug. Drugs that function in this manner are known as **prodrugs** (see Section 9.8). For example, the bacteriacide prontosil, discovered in 1935, is not active but is metabolized *in situ* to the antibacterial sulphanilamide.

Prontosil   Sulphanilamide

2.7.1.3 Metabolism

Drug metabolism is the biotransformation of the drug into other compounds referred to as **metabolites**. These biotransformations occur mainly in the liver but they can also occur in blood and other organs such as the brain, lungs and kidneys (see Section 9.3). Metabolism of a drug usually reduces the concentration of that drug in the systemic circulation, which normally leads to either a lowering or a complete suppression of the pharmacological action and toxic effects of that drug. Exceptions are prodrugs (see Section 9.8), such as prontosil, where metabolism produces the active form of the drug.

Metabolism usually involves more than one route and results in the formation of a sucession of metabolites (Figure 2.5). Each of these metabolites may have a different or similar activity to the parent drug (see Section 9.2). Consequently, the activities of all the metabolities of a drug must be considered in the development of a potential drug. Metabolities are frequently more water soluble than their parent drug and because of this are usually excreted in the urine.

2.7.1.4 Elimination

Elimination is the collective term used for metabolic and excretion processes that **irreversibly** remove a drug from the body during its journey to its site of action. It reduces the medical effect of the drug by reducing its concentration at

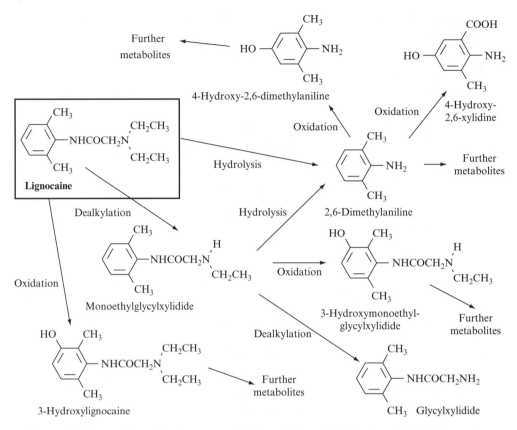

Figure 2.5 An outline of the known metabolic pathways of the local anaesthetic lignocaine

its site of action. A slow elimination process can result in a build-up of the drug concentration in the body. This may benefit the patient in that the dose required to maintain the therapeutic effect can be reduced, which in turn reduces the chances of unwanted side effects. Conversely, the rapid elimination of a drug means that the patient has to receive either increased doses, with a greater risk of toxic side effects, or more frequent doses, which carries more risk of under- or over-dosing. The main excretion route for drugs and their metabolites is through the kidney in solution in the urine. However, a significant number of drugs and their metabolic products are also excreted via the bowel in the faeces.

Drugs are eliminated in the kidneys by either **glomerular filtration** or **tubular secretion**. However, some of the species lost by these processes are reabsorbed by a recycling process known as **tubular reabsorption**. Tubular reabsorption is a process normally employed in returning compounds such as water, amino acids, salts and glucose that are important to the well-being of the body from the urine to the circulatory system, but it will also return drug molecules. The reabsorption of acidic and basic drugs is reduced if the pH favours salt formation as charged molecules are not readily transported across membranes (see Appendices 3 and 5).

Elimination occurs in the liver by **biliary clearance**, very large molecules being metabolized to smaller compounds before being excreted. However, a fraction of some of the excreted drugs is reabsorbed through the **enterohepatic cycle**. This reabsorption can be reduced by the use of suitable substances in the dosage form, for example, the ion exchange resin cholestyramine is used to reduce cholesterol levels by preventing its reabsorption.

2.7.2 Bioavailability of a drug

The bioavailability of a drug is defined as the fraction of the dose of a drug that is found in general circulation (see Section 8.5). It is influenced by such factors as ADME. Bioavailability is not constant but varies with the body's physiological condition.

2.7.3 The pharmacodynamic phase

Pharmacodynamics is concerned with the result of the interaction of drug and body at its site of action, that is, what the drug does to the body. It is now known that a drug is most effective when its shape and electron distribution, that is, its **stereoelectronic structure**, is complementary to the stereoelectronic structure of the active site or receptor.

The role of the medicinal chemist is to design and synthesize a drug structure that has the maximum beneficial effects with a minimum of toxic side effects. This design has to take into account the stereoelectronic characteristics of the target active or receptor site and also such factors as the drug's stability *in situ*, its polarity and its relative solubilities in aqueous media and lipids. The stereo-chemistry of the drug is particularly important, as stereoisomers often have different biological effects, which range from inactive to highly toxic (see Table 2.1).

Table 2.1 Variations in the biological activities of stereoisomers

First stereoisomer	Second stereoisomer	Example
Active	Activity of same type and potency	The R and S isomers of the antimalarial chloroquine have equal potencies.
Active	Activity the same type but weaker	The E isomer of diethylstilbesterol, an estrogen is only 7% as active as the Z isomer
Active	Activity of a different type	S-Ketamine is an anaesthetic R-Ketamine has little anaesthetic action but is a psychotic
Active	No activity	S-α-Methyldopa is a hypertensive drug but the R isomer is inactive.
Active	Active but different side effects	Thalidomide: the S isomer is a sedative and has teratogenic side effects. The R isomer is also a sedative but has no teratogenic activity.

2.8   Questions

(1)   Explain the meaning of the terms (a) lead compound, (b) excipient, (c) parenteral administration, (d) pharmacophore and (e) prodrug.

(2)   State the general factors that need to be considered when designing a drug.

(3)   Distinguish between parenteral and enteral routes of administration.

(4)   Define the terms pharmacokinetic phase and pharmacodynamic phase in the context of drug action. List the main general factors that affect these phases.

(5)   The drug amphetamine ($PhCH_2CH(NH_2)CH_3$ binds to the protein albumin in the blood stream. Predict how a reduction in pH would be expected to influence this binding. Albumin is negatively charged at pH 7.4 and electrically neutral at pH 5.0.

(6)   Discuss the general effects that stereoisomers could have on the activity of a drug.

3 An Introduction to Drug Discovery

3.1 Introduction

Drug discovery is part luck and part structured investigation. At the begining of the 19th century it was largely carried out by individuals but it now requires teamwork, the members of the team being specialists in various fields, such as medicine, biochemistry, chemistry, computerized molecular modelling, pharmaceutics, pharmacology, microbiology, toxicology, physiology and pathology. This chapter outlines a general approach to drug discovery by design. It also introduces the stereochemical and water solubility factors that should be taken into account when selecting a structure for a lead compound.

The approach to drug design depends on the objectives of the design team. These objectives will normally require a detailed assessment of the pathology of the disease and in some cases basic biochemical research will be necessary before initiating a drug design investigation (Figure 3.1). The information obtained is used by the team to decide what intervention would be most likely to bring about the desired result. Once the point of intervention has been selected, the team has to propose a structure for a lead compound that could possibly bring about the required change. This frequently requires an extensive literature and database search to identify compounds found in the organism (**endogenous compounds**) and compounds that are not found in the organism (**exogenous compounds**) that have some biological effect at the intervention site. Molecular modelling techniques (see Chapter 5) are sometimes used to help the team reach a decision. In many cases, a number of structures are found to be suitable, but the expense of producing drugs dictates that the team has to choose only one or two of these compounds to either act as the lead or to be the inspiration for the lead compound. The final selection depends on the experience of the team.

Fundamentals of Medicinal Chemistry, Edited by Gareth Thomas
© 2003 John Wiley & Sons, Ltd
ISBN 0 470 84306 3 (Hbk), ISBN 0 470 84307 1 (pbk)

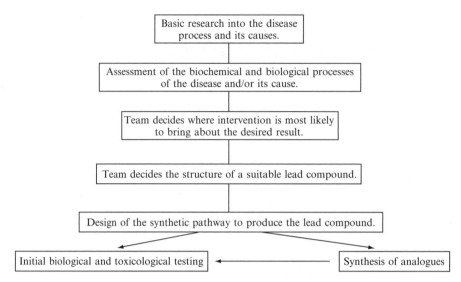

Figure 3.1   The general steps in the design of a new drug

A more random approach to discovering a lead is the combinatorial chemistry approach (see Chapter 6). This uses a simultaneous multiple synthesis technique to produce large numbers of potential leads. These potential leads are subjected to rapid high throughput biological screening to identify the most active lead compounds. Once identified, these lead compounds are subject to further development.

Once the structure of the proposed lead has been agreed, it becomes the responsibility of the medicinal chemist to devise a synthetic route and prepare a sample of this compound for testing. Once synthesized, the compound undergoes initial pharmacological and toxicological testing. The results of these tests enable the team to decide whether it is profitable to continue development by preparing analogues (Figure 3.1), since it is unlikely that the lead compound itself will be suitable for use as a drug. The usual scenario is to prepare a series of analogues, measure their activity and correlate the results to determine the structure with optimum activity. This analysis may make use of SARs (see Chapter 4), QSARs (see Chapter 4.), computational chemistry (see Chapter 5) and combinatorial chemistry (see Chapter 6) to help discover the nature of this structure.

The selection of a lead compound and the development of a synthetic pathway for its preparation (see Chapters 10 and 11) is not the only consideration at the start of an investigation. Researchers must also devise suitable *in vivo* and *in vitro* tests to assess the activity and toxicity of the compounds produced. There is no point in carrying out an expensive synthetic procedure if at the end of the day it is impossible to test the product.

3.2   Stereochemistry and drug design

It is now well established that the shape of a molecule is normally one of the most important factors affecting drug activity. Consequently, the overall shape of the structure of a molecule is an important consideration when designing an analogue. Some structural features impose a considerable degree of rigidity on a structure, whilst others make the structure more flexible. Other structures give rise to stereoisomers, which can exhibit different potencies, types of activity and unwanted side effects (see Table 2.1). This means that it is necessary to pharmacologically evaluate individual stereoisomers and racemates. Consequently, one must take into account all these stereochemical features when proposing structures for potential leads and analogues. However, the extent to which one can exploit these structural features will depend on our knowledge of the structure and biochemistry of the target biological system.

3.2.1   Structurally rigid groups

Groups that are structurally rigid are unsaturated groups of all types and saturated ring systems (Figure 3.2). The former includes esters and amides as well as aliphatic conjugated systems, aromatic and heteroaromatic ring systems. The binding of these rigid structures to a target site can give information about the shape of that site as well as the nature of the interaction between the site and the ligand. Furthermore, the fact that the structure is rigid means it may be replaced by alternative rigid structures of a similar size and shape to form analogues, which may have different binding characteristics and possibly as a result a different activity or potency (see sections 2.3 and 4.3.2).

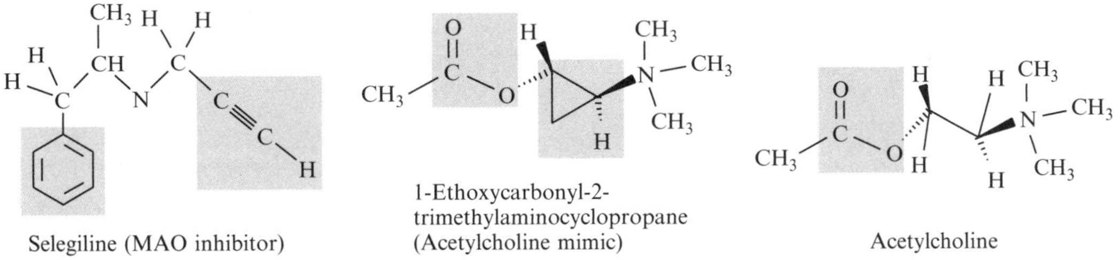

Selegiline (MAO inhibitor)

1-Ethoxycarbonyl-2-
trimethylaminocyclopropane
(Acetylcholine mimic)

Acetylcholine

Figure 3.2   Examples of structural groups that impose a rigid shape on sections of a molecule. The shaded areas represent the rigid sections of the molecule

3.2.2 Conformation

Early work in the 1950s and early 1960s by Schueler and Archer suggested that the flexibility of the structures of both ligands and receptors accounted for the same ligand being able to bind to different sub-types of a receptor (see Appendix 4). Archer also concluded that a ligand appeared to assume different conformations when it bound to the different sub-types of a receptor. For example, acetylcholine exhibits both muscarinic and nicotinic activity. Archer *et al.* suggested that the muscarinic activity was due to the *anti* or staggered conformation, whilst the nicotinic activity was due to the *syn* or eclipsed form (Figure 3.3).

The main methods of introducing conformational restrictions are by using either bulky substituents, unsaturated structures or ring systems. Ring systems are usually the most popular choice (Figure 3.4). In all cases, the structures used must be chosen with care, because there will always be the possibility that steric hindrance will prevent the binding of the analogue to the target. However, if sufficient information is available, molecular modelling (see section 5.5) can be of considerable assistance in the choice of structures.

3.2.3 Configuration

Configurational centres impose a rigid shape on sections of the molecule in which they occur. However, their presence gives rise to geometric and optical isomerism. Since these stereoisomers have different shapes, biologically active stereoisomers will often exhibit differences in their potencies and/or activities (Table 2.1). These pharmacological variations are particularly likely when a chiral centre is located in a critical position in the structure of the molecule. The consequence of these differences is that it is now necessary to make and test separately all the individual stereoisomers of a drug.

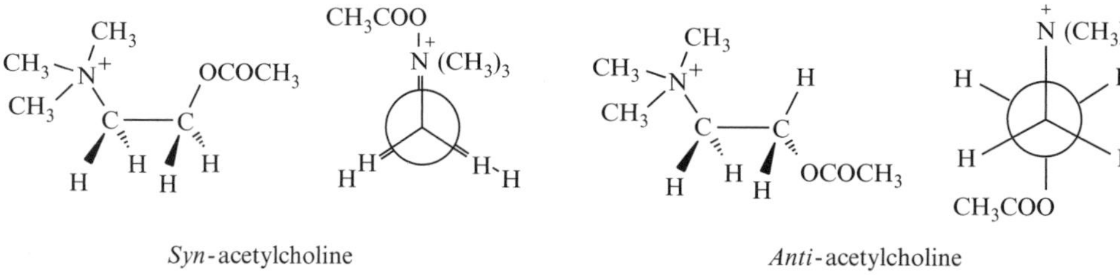

Syn-acetylcholine   *Anti*-acetylcholine

Figure 3.3 *Syn* and *anti* conformers of acetylcholine and 2-tropanyl ethanoate methiodides

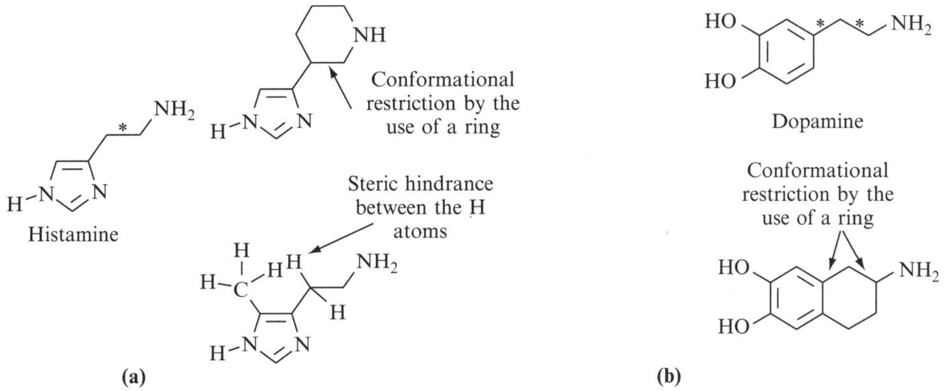

Figure 3.4 Examples of the use of conformational restrictions to produce analogues of (a) histamine and (b) dopamine. Bonds marked * can exhibit free rotation and form numerous conformers

As well as an effect on the activity, different stereoisomers will also exhibit differences in other physiochemical properties, such as absorption, metabolism and elimination. For example, (−)norgestrel is absorbed at twice the rate of (+)norgestrel through buccal and vaginal membranes. The plasma half life of S-indacrinone is 2–5 hours whilst the value for the R isomer is 10–12 hours.

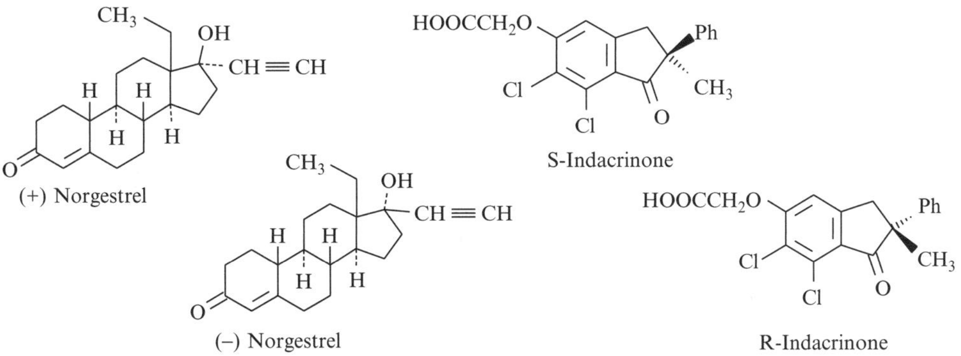

3.3 Solubility and drug design

The relative solubilities of drugs in the aqueous media and lipid tissues of the body play a major part in their absorption and transport to their sites of action.

To pass through a membrane (see Appendices 3 and 5) a drug must usually exhibit a reasonable degree of both water and lipid solubility (see section 2.7.1). An appropriate degree of water solubility will often improve drug distribution within the circulatory system as well as drug action.

3.3.1 The importance of water solubility

A drug's solubility and behaviour in water is particularly important since the cells in our bodies normally contain about 65% water. In living matter, water acts as an inert solvent, a dispersing medium for colloidal solutions and as a nucleophilic reagent in numerous biological reactions. Furthermore, hydrogen bonding and hydrophobic interactions in water influence the conformations of biological macromolecules, which in turn affects their biological behaviour. It also makes drug toxicity testing and bioavailability evaluation as well as clinical application easier. This means that there is usually a need to design a reasonable degree of water solubility into the structure of a new drug early in the development of that drug.

Drugs administered orally as a solid or in suspension have to dissolve in the aqueous gastric fluid (*dissolution*) before they can be absorbed and transported *via* the systemic circulation to their site of action. The rate and extent of dissolution of a drug is a major factor in controlling the absorption of that drug. This is because the concentration of the drug in the fluid in the gut lumen is one of the main factors governing the transfer of the drug through the membranes (see Appendix 5) of the gastrointestinal tract (GI tract). The rate of dissolution depends on the surface area of the solid, which is dependent on both the physical nature of the dosage form of the drug and the chemical structure of the drug. However, the extent of dissolution depends only on the drug's solubility, which depends on the chemical structure of the drug. The dosage form is a formulation problem that is normally beyond the remit of the medicinal chemist, but the design of the structure of lead compounds with regard to solubility is within the realm of the medicinal chemist.

Once the drug has entered the circulatory system, either by absorption or by direct administration, its water solubility will influence its ease of transport to the body compartments available to that drug. Drugs that are sparingly soluble in water may be deposited *en route* to their site of action, which can clog up blood vessels and damage organs. For example, many sulphonamides, such as sulphamethoxazole, tend to crystallize in the kidney, which may result in serious liver and kidney damage. Water solubility also affects the ease of drug transport through membranes (see section 4.4.1).

Pyrantel embonate

(Embonate)

The sulphonamide group

Sulphamethoxazole (antibacterial)

Although a reasonable degree of water solubility is normally regarded as an essential requirement for a potential drug, it is possible to utilize poor water solubility in drug action and therapy. For example, pyrantel embonate, which is used to treat pinworm and hookworm infestations of the GI tract, is insoluble in water. This poor water solubility coupled with the polar nature of the salt (see section 2.1.1) means that the drug is poorly absorbed from the gut and so the greater part of the dose is retained in the GI tract, the drug's site of action. The low water solubility of a drug can also be used to produce drug depots, chewable dosage forms and mask bitter tasting drugs, because taste depends on the substance forming an aqueous solution.

The importance of water solubility in drug action means that one of the medicinal chemist's development targets for a new drug is to develop analogues that have the required degree of water solubility.

3.4 Solubility and drug structure

The solubility of a compound depends on its degree of solvation in the solvent. Structural features in a solute molecule that improve the degree of solvation will result in a more soluble solute. Consequently, the water solubility of an organic compound depends on the number and nature of the polar groups in its structure as well as the size of its carbon–hydrogen skeleton. In general, the higher the ratio of polar groups to the total number of carbon atoms in the structure the more water soluble the compound. Furthermore, aromatic compounds tend to be less soluble than the corresponding nonaromatic compounds. Using these general rules, it is possible to assess the relative solubilities of compounds with similar carbon–hydrogen skeletons. However, the more complex the structure, the less accurate these assessments.

The water solubility of a lead compound can be improved by three general methods: salt formation (see section 3.5), by incorporating water solubilizing groups into its structure (see section 3.6), especially those that can hydrogen bond with water, and the use of special dosage forms, a discussion of the latter being beyond the scope of this text. In salt formation, the activity of the drug is normally unchanged although its potency may be different. However, when new structural groups are incorporated into the structure of a drug the activity of the drug could be changed. Consequently, it will be necessary to carry out a full trial programme on the new analogue. Both these modifications can be costly processes if they have to be carried out at a late stage in drug development. The use of specialized dosage forms does not usually need extensive additions to the trials programme but these formulation methods are only suitable for use with some drugs.

The structural factors controlling a compound's lipid solubility are the opposite of those responsible for a compound's water solubility. Consequently, lipid solubility may be improved by replacing polar groups by nonpolar structures or groups that are significantly less polar in nature.

3.5   Salt formation

Salt formation usually improves the water solubility of acidic and basic drugs because the salts of these drugs dissociate in water to produce hydrated ions:

$$salt \rightleftharpoons cation + anion$$

Hydrogen and hydroxide ions can disturb this equilibrium if they combine with the appropriate cation or anion to form less soluble acids or bases. Consequently, the pH of the biological fluid may affect the solubility of a drug and, as a result, its activity. In general, increasing the hydrophilic nature of the salt should increase its water solubility. However, there are numerous exceptions to this generalization, and each salt should be treated on its merits.

Acidic drugs are usually converted to their metallic or amino salts, whilst the salts of organic acids are normally used for basic drugs (Table 3.1).

The degree of water solubility of a salt will depends on the structure of the acid or base (see section 3.4) used to form the salt. For example, acids and bases whose structures contain water solubilizing groups will form salts with a higher water solubility than compounds that do not contain these groups (Figure 3.5). However, if a drug is too water soluble, it will not dissolve in lipids and so will not usually be readily transported through lipid membranes (Appendix 5). This normally results in either its activity being reduced, or the time for its onset of action being increased. It should also be noted that the

Table 3.1   Examples of the acids and bases used to form the salts of drugs

Anions and anion sources	Cations and cation sources
Ethanoic acid – ethanoate (CH_3COO^-)	Sodium – sodium ion (Na^+)
Citric acid – citrate (see Figure 3.5)	Calcium – calcium ion (Ca^{2+})
Lactic acid – lactate (see Figure 3.5)	Zinc – zinc ion (Zn^{2+})
Tartaric acid – tartrate (see Figure 3.5)	Diethanolamine – $R_2NH_2^+$ (see Figure 3.5)
Hydrochloric acid – chloride (Cl^-)	N-Methylglucamine – $RNH_2^+CH_3$ (see Figure 3.5)
Sulphuric acid – sulphate (SO_4^{2-})	2-Aminoethanol ($HN_2CH_2CH_2OH$) – RNH_3^+
Sulphuric acid – hydrogen sulphate (HSO_4^-)	

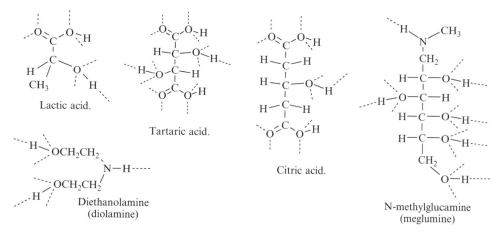

Figure 3.5   Examples of the structures of acids and bases whose structures contain water solubilizing groups. The possible positions of hydrogen bonds are shown by the dashed lines------; lone pairs are omitted for clarity. At room temperature it is highly unlikely that all the possible hydrogen bonds will be formed. *Note:* hydrogen bonds are not shown for the acidic protons of the acids as these protons are donated to the base on salt formation. Similarly, no hydrogen bonds are shown for the lone pairs of the amino groups, because these lone pairs accept a proton in salt formation

presence of a high concentration of chloride ions in the stomach will reduce the solubility of sparingly soluble chloride salts because of the common ion effect.

3.6   The incorporation of water solubilizing groups in a structure

The discussion of the introduction of water solubilizing groups into the structure of a lead compound can be conveniently broken down into four general areas:

1. the type of group introduced;

2. whether the introduction is reversible or irreversible;

3. the position of incorporation and

4. the chemical route of introduction.

3.6.1   The type of group

The incorporation of polar groups, such as the alcohol, amine, amide, carboxylic acid, sulphonic acid and phosphorus oxyacid groups, which either ionize or are capable of relatively strong intermolecular forces of attraction with water (hydrogen bonding), will usually result in analogues with an increased water solubility. Acidic and basic groups are particularly useful, since these groups can be used to form salts (see section 3.5), which would give a wider range of dosage forms for the final product. However, the formation of zwitterions by the introduction of either an acid group into a structure containing a base or a base group into a structure containing an acid group can reduce water solubility. Introduction of weakly polar groups, such as carboxylic acid esters, aryl halides and alkyl halides, will not significantly improve water solubility and can result in enhanced lipid solubility. In all cases, the degree of solubility obtained by the incorporation cannot be accurately predicted since it also depends on other factors. Consequently, the type of group introduced is generally selected on the basis of previous experience.

The incorporation of acidic residues into a lead structure is less likely to change the type of activity, but it can result in the analogue exhibiting haemolytic properties. Furthermore, the introduction of an aromatic acid group usually results in anti-inflammatory activity, whilst carboxylic acids with an alpha functional group may act as chelating agents. Basic water solubilizing groups have a tendency to change the mode of action, since bases often interfere with neurotransmitters and biological processes involving amines. However, their incorporation does mean that the analogue can be formulated as a wide variety of acid salts. Nonionizable groups do not have the disadvantages of acidic and basic groups.

3.6.2   Reversibly and irreversibly attached groups

The type of group selected also depends on the degree of permanency required. Groups that are bound directly to the carbon skeleton of the lead compound by less reactive C–C, C–O and C–N bonds are likely to be irreversibly attached to the lead structure. Groups that are linked to the lead by ester, amide, phosphate, sulphate and glycosidic links are more likely to be metabolized from the resulting analogue to reform the parent lead compound as the analogue is transferred from its point of administration to its site of action. Compounds with this type of solubilizing group are acting as prodrugs (see section 9.8) and so their activity is more likely to be the same as the parent lead compound. However, the rate of loss of the solubilizing group will depend on the nature of the transfer route, and this could affect the activity of the drug.

3.6.3 The position of the water solubilizing group

In order to preserve the type of activity exhibited by the lead compound, the water solubilizing group should be attached to a part of the structure that is not involved in the drug–receptor interaction. Consequently, the route used to introduce a new water solubilizing group and its position in the lead structure will depend on the relative reactivities of the pharmacophore and the rest of the molecule. The reagents used to introduce the new water solubilizing group should be chosen on the basis that they do not react with, or in close proximity to, the pharmacophore. This will reduce the possibility of the new group affecting the relevant drug–receptor interactions.

3.6.4 Methods of introduction

Water solubilizing groups are best introduced at the begining of a drug synthesis, although they may be introduced at any stage. Introduction at the begining avoids the problem of a later introduction changing the type and/or nature of the drug–receptor interaction. A wide variety of routes may be used to introduce a water solubilizing group; the one selected will depend on the type of group being introduced and the chemical nature of the target structure (Figures 3.6 and 3.7). Many of these routes require the use of protecting agents to prevent unwanted reactions of either the water solubilizing group or the lead structure.

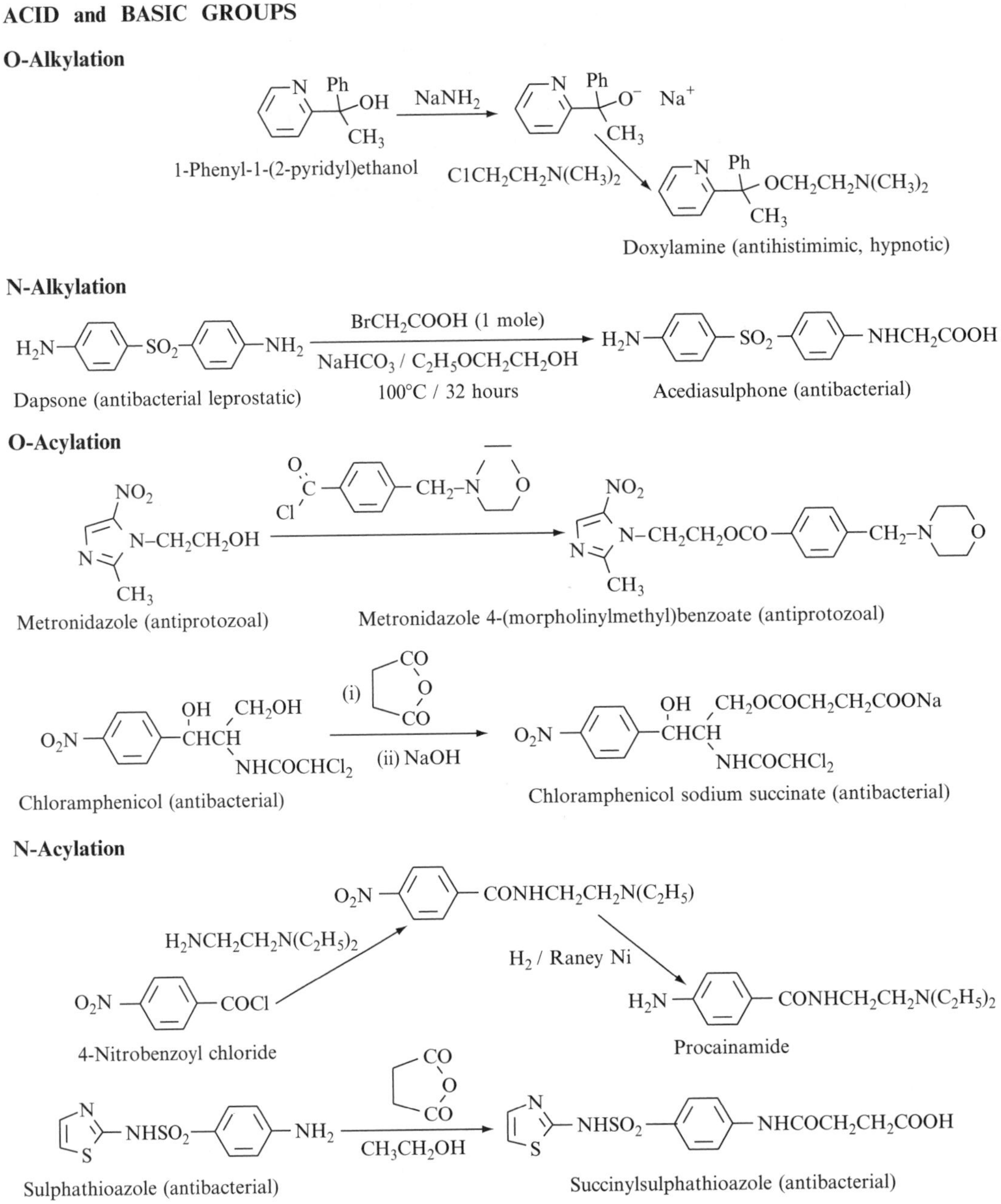

ACID and BASIC GROUPS

O-Alkylation

1-Phenyl-1-(2-pyridyl)ethanol

$\xrightarrow{\text{NaNH}_2}$

$\text{ClCH}_2\text{CH}_2\text{N(CH}_3)_2$

Doxylamine (antihistimimic, hypnotic)

N-Alkylation

H_2N—⟨ ⟩—SO_2—⟨ ⟩—NH_2 $\xrightarrow[\substack{\text{NaHCO}_3 / \text{C}_2\text{H}_5\text{OCH}_2\text{CH}_2\text{OH} \\ 100°\text{C} / 32 \text{ hours}}]{\text{BrCH}_2\text{COOH (1 mole)}}$ H_2N—⟨ ⟩—SO_2—⟨ ⟩—$NHCH_2COOH$

Dapsone (antibacterial leprostatic)   Acediasulphone (antibacterial)

O-Acylation

Metronidazole (antiprotozoal)   Metronidazole 4-(morpholinylmethyl)benzoate (antiprotozoal)

Chloramphenicol (antibacterial) $\xrightarrow[\text{(ii) NaOH}]{\text{(i)}}$ Chloramphenicol sodium succinate (antibacterial)

N-Acylation

O_2N—⟨ ⟩—$COCl$ $\xrightarrow{H_2NCH_2CH_2N(C_2H_5)_2}$ O_2N—⟨ ⟩—$CONHCH_2CH_2N(C_2H_5)$

4-Nitrobenzoyl chloride

$\xrightarrow{H_2 / \text{Raney Ni}}$ H_2N—⟨ ⟩—$CONHCH_2CH_2N(C_2H_5)_2$

Procainamide

Sulphathioazole (antibacterial) $\xrightarrow{CH_3CH_2OH}$ Succinylsulphathioazole (antibacterial)

Figure 3.6 Examples of water solubilizing structures and the routes used to introduce them into the lead structures. O-alkylation, N-alkylation, O-acylation and N-acylation reactions are used to introduce both acidic and basic groups. Acetylation methods use both the appropriate acid chloride and anhydride.

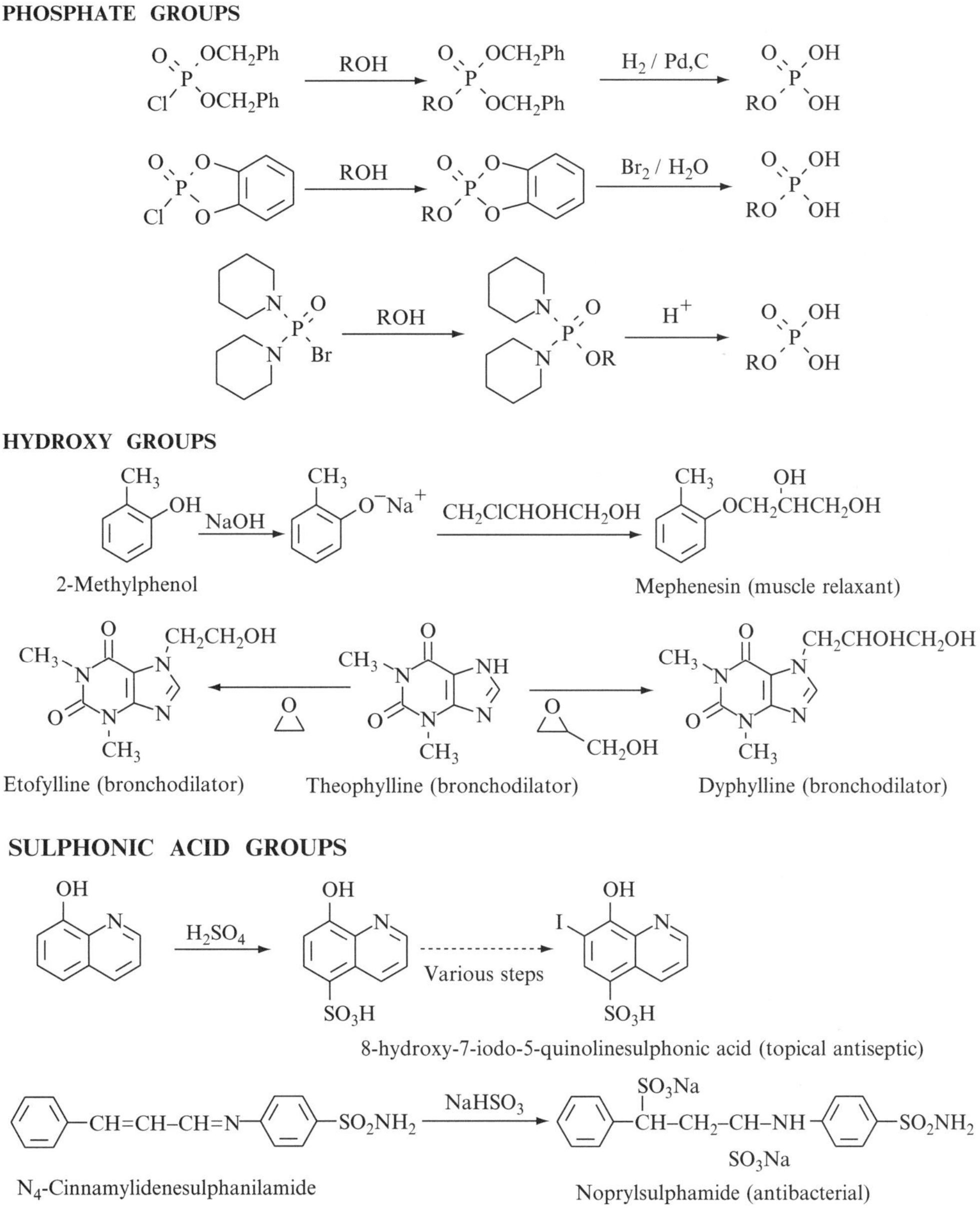
PHOSPHATE GROUPS
ROH
H2 / Pd,C
Br2 / H2O
H+
HYDROXY GROUPS
NaOH
CH2ClCHOHCH2OH
2-Methylphenol
Mephenesin (muscle relaxant)
Etofylline (bronchodilator)
Theophylline (bronchodilator)
Dyphylline (bronchodilator)
SULPHONIC ACID GROUPS
H2SO4
Various steps
8-hydroxy-7-iodo-5-quinolinesulphonic acid (topical antiseptic)
NaHSO3
N4-Cinnamylidenesulphanilamide
Noprylsulphamide (antibacterial)

Figure 3.7 Examples of water solubilizing structures and the routes used to introduce them into lead structures. Phosphate acid halides have been used to introduce phosphate groups into lead structures. The hydroxy groups of the acid halide must normally be protected by a suitable protecting group. These protecting groups are removed in the final stage of the synthesis to reveal the water solubilizing phosphate ester. Structures containing hydroxy groups have been introduced by reaction of the corresponding monochlorinated hydrin and the use of suitable epoxides amongst other methods. Sulphonic acid groups may be introduced by either direct sulphonation or the addition of bisulphite to reactive $C = C$ bonds amongst other methods

3.7 Questions

(1) Outline the general steps in the discovery of a new drug.

(2) Outline by means of suitable examples the significance of (i) structurally rigid groups, (ii) conformations and (iii) configuration on the design of new drugs.

(3) Explain why water solubility is an important factor in drug design.

(4) List the structural features that would indicate whether a compound is likely to be reasonably water soluble. Illustrate the answer by reference to suitable examples.

(5) Suggest general methods by which the water solubility of a compound could be improved without affecting its type of biological action.

(6) Suggest, by means of chemical equations, one route for the introduction of each of (i) an acid residue and (ii) a basic residue into the structure of 4-hydroxybenzenesulphonamide when the sulphonamide group acts as the pharmacophore in this compound.

4 The SAR and QSAR approaches to drug design

4.1 Structure–activity relationships (SARS)

Compounds with similar structures to a pharmacologically active drug are often themselves biologically active. This activity may be either similar to that of the original compound but different in potency and unwanted side effects or completely different to that exhibited by the original compound. These structurally related activities are commonly referred to as **structure–activity relationships** (SARS). A study of the structure–activity relationships of a lead compound and its analogues may be used to determine the parts of the structure of the lead compound that are responsible for both its beneficial biological activity, that is, its **pharmacophore,** and also its unwanted side effects. This information may be used to develop a new drug that has increased activity, a different activity from an existing drug and fewer unwanted side effects.

Structure–activity relationships are usually determined by making minor changes to the structure of a lead to produce analogues (see section 2.3) and assessing the effect these structural changes have on biological activity. The investigation of numerous lead compounds and their analogues has made it possible to make some broad generalizations about the biological effects of specific types of structural change. These changes may be conveniently classified as changing

1. the size and shape of the carbon skeleton (see section 4.2),

2. the nature and degree of substitution (see section 4.3), and

3. the stereochemistry of the lead (see section 3.2).

Fundamentals of Medicinal Chemistry, Edited by Gareth Thomas
© 2003 John Wiley & Sons, Ltd
ISBN 0 470 84306 3 (Hbk), ISBN 0 470 84307 1 (pbk)

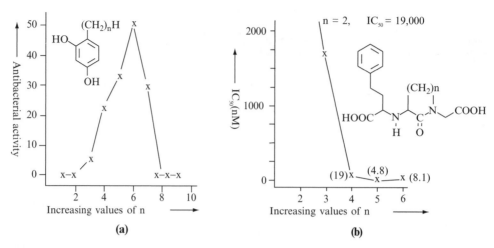

Figure 4.1 Examples of the variation of response curves with increasing numbers of inserted methylene groups. (a) A study by Dohme *et al.* on the variation of antibacterial activity of 4-alkyl substituted resorcinols. (b) Inhibition of ACE by enalaprilat analogues (Thorsett). The figures in brackets are the IC_{50} values for that analogue

The selection of the changes required to produce analogues of a particular lead is made by considering the activities of compounds with similar structures and also the possible chemistry and biochemistry of the intended analogue. It is believed that structural changes that result in analogues with increased lipid character may exhibit either increased activity because of better membrane penetration (Figure 4.1(a); $n = 3$–6) or reduced activity because of a reduction in their water solubility (Figure 4.1(b)). However, whatever the change, its effect on water solubility, transport through membranes, receptor binding, and metabolism and other pharmacokinetic properties of the analogue should be considered as far as is possible before embarking on what could be an expensive synthesis. Furthermore, changing the structure of the lead compound could result in an analogue that is too big to fit its intended target site. Computer assisted molecular modelling (see Chapter 5) can alleviate this problem, provided that the structure of the target is known or can be simulated with some degree of accuracy. However, it is emphasized that although it is possible to predict the effect of structural changes there will be numerous exceptions to the predictions, and so all analogues must be synthesized and tested.

4.2   Changing size and shape

The shapes and sizes of molecules can be modified in a variety of ways, such as changing the number of methylene groups in chains and rings, increasing or decreasing the degree of unsaturation and introducing or removing a ring system (Table 4.1). These types of structural change usually result in analogues that exhibit either a different potency or a different type of activity to the lead.

4.3   Introduction of new substituents

The new substituents may either occupy a previously unsubstituted position in the lead compound (see section 4.3.1) or replace an existing substituent (see section 4.3.2). Each new substituent will impart its own characteristic chemical, pharmacokinetic and pharmacodynamic properties to the analogue. Over the years, a great deal of information has been collected about the changes caused to these properties of a lead compound when a new substituent is incorporated into its structure. As a result, it is possible to generalize about some of the changes caused by the introduction of a particular group into a structure (see Table 4.2). However, the choice of substituent will ultimately depend on the properties that the development team decide to enhance in an attempt to meet their objectives. Moreover, it should be realized that the practical results of such a structural change will often be different from the theoretical predictions.

4.3.1   The introduction of a group in an unsubstituted position

The incorporation of any group will always result in analogues with a different size and shape to the lead compound. In addition, it may introduce a chiral centre, which will result in the formation of stereoisomers, which may or may not have different pharmacological activities (Table 2.1). Alternatively, it may impose conformation restrictions on some of the bonds in the analogue (Figure 4.2).

The introduction of a new group may result in an increased rate of metabolism, a reduction in the rate of metabolism or an alternative route for metabolism (see Chapter 9). These changes could also change the duration of action and the nature of any side effects. For example, mono- and diortho-methylation with respect to the phenolic hydroxy group of paracetamol produces analogues with

Table 4.1 Examples of the ways in which the size and shape of the carbon skeletons of lead compounds may be changed to produce new analogues

Change	Notes	Example, the lead compound is given in square brackets([ ])
The number of methylene (CH₂) groups in a chain or ring.	Increasing the number of CH₂ groups in a *chain* can lead to micelle formation which can reduce drug activity (Fig. 4.1). Changing the number of CH₂ groups in a *ring* may lead to a change in activity.	Chlorpromazine (Antipsychotic) Clomipramine (Antidepressant)
The degree of unsaturation.	Introduction of a double bond increases the rigidity of the structure and in some cases the possibility of E and Z isomers. The reduction of double bonds makes the structure more flexible.	Cortisol (Anti-inflammatory) Prednisone (Potency × 30) *Note.* No E isomer is possible in this example.
Addition or removal of a ring.	Introduction of a ring may result in the filling of a hydrophobic pocket in the target, which might improve the binding of the drug to its target.	3-(3,4-Dimethoxy phenyl)-butyrolactam (Antidepressant) Rolipram (Potency × 10)
	The incorporation of larger ring systems may be used to produce analogues that are resistant to enzymic attack.	Benzylpenicillin (not β-lactamase resistant) Diphenicillin (β-lactamase resistant)
	Removal of ring systems has been used to produce analogues of naturally occuring active compounds.	Morphine (Narcotic analgesic) Pethidine (Narcotic analgesic)

Table 4.2 Examples of some of the groups commonly used as new substituents in the production of analogues

Group	Effect on lipophilic character	Likely change in solubility (see sections 3.3 and 3.4)	Notes
Methyl	Increased lipophilic character	Decreased water solubility. Increased lipid solubility.	Improves ease of absorption but makes its release from biological membranes more difficult. Can lead to changes in the nature and rate of metabolism. Larger alkyl groups will have similar effects.
Fluorine and chlorine	Increased lipophilic character	Decreased water solubility. Increased lipid solubility.	Used to improve ease of penetration of cell membranes. However, there is an undesireable tendency for halogenated drugs to accumulate in lipid tissues. CF_3 groups are sometimes used to replace Cl groups as these groups are of a similar size.
Hydroxy	Decreased lipophilic character	Increased water solubility. Decreased lipid solubility.	Provides a new centre for hydrogen, which could influence the binding of the drug to the target site. The presence of the hydroxy group could result in an increase in the rate of elimination of the drug by a new metabolic pathway and/or excretion.
Amino groups	Decreased lipophilic character	Increased water solubility due to salt formation. Decreased lipid solubility.	Provides a new centre for hydrogen bonding, which could influence the binding of the drug to the target site. The incorporation of aromatic amines is avoided as they are often toxic and/or carcinogenic.
Carboxylic and sulphonic groups	Decreased lipophilic character	Increased water solubility due to salt formation. Decreased lipid solubility	Water solubility may be enhanced by *in vivo* salt formation. Introduction usually increases the ease of elimination. Carboxylic acid group introduction into small lead molecules may change the type of activity of the analogue whilst sulphonic acid group incorporation does not normally change the type of activity.

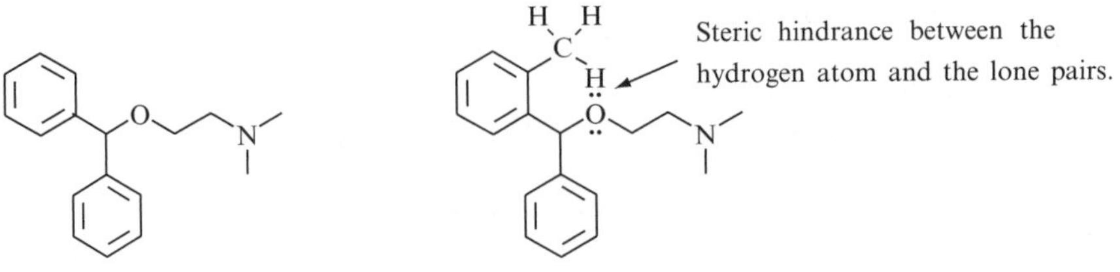

Diphenhydramine   o-Methyl analogue

Figure 4.2 Harmes *et al.* suggest that the lack of antihistamine activity in the ortho-methyl analogue of diphenyhydramine is due to the ortho-methyl group restricting rotation about the C–O bond. It is believed that this prevents the molecule from adopting the conformation necessary for antihistamine activity

reduced hepatotoxicity. It is believed that this reduction is due to the methyl groups preventing metabolic hydroxylation of these ortho positions.

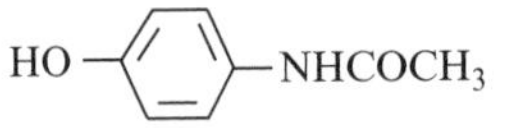

Paracetamol 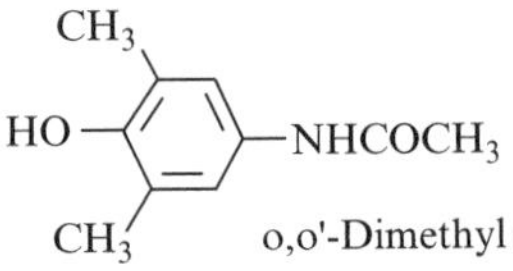   o,o'-Dimethyl analogue of paracetamol

The position of substitution is critical. In one position the new group will lead to an enhancement of activity, while in another position it will result in a reduction of activity. For example, the antihypertensive clonidine with its o,o'-dichloro substitution is more potent than its m,p-dichloro analogue (Figure 4.3).

4.3.2 The introduction of a group by replacing an existing group

Analogues formed by replacing an existing group by a new group may exhibit the general stereochemical and metabolic changes outlined in section 4.3.1. The choice of group will depend on the objectives of the design team. It is often made using the concept of *isosteres*. Isosteres are groups that exhibit some similarities

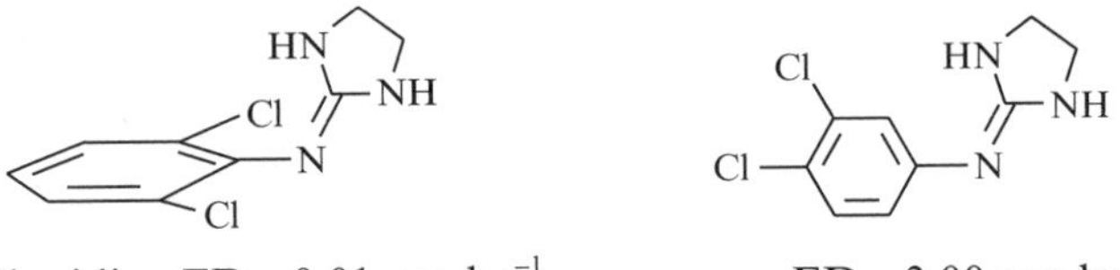

Clonidine ED_{20} 0.01 mg kg^{-1} ED_{20} 3.00 mg kg^{-1}

Figure 4.3 Clonidine and its m,p-dichloro analogue. It is believed that the bulky chloro groups impose a conformation restriction on clonidine, which probably accounts for its greater activity

Table 4.3 Examples of isosteres. Each horizontal row represents a group of structures that are isosteric. Classical isosteres were originally defined by Erlenmeyer as atoms, ions and molecules with identical shells of electrons. Bioisosteres are groups with similar structures that usually exhibit similar biological activities

Classical isosteres	Bioisosteres		
$-CH_3$, $-NH_2$, $-OH$, $-F$, $-Cl$			
$-Cl$, $-SH$ $-PH_2$			
$-Br$, Isopropyl 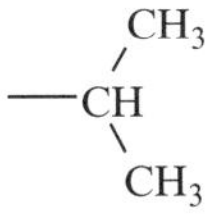			
$-CH_2-$, $-NH-$, $-O-$, $-S-$			
$-COCH_2R$, $-CONHR$, $-COOR$, $-COSR$			
$-HC=$, $-N=$			
In rings: $-CH=CH-$, $-S-$ $-O-$, $-S-$, $-CH_2-$, $-NH-$ $-CH=$, $-N-$			

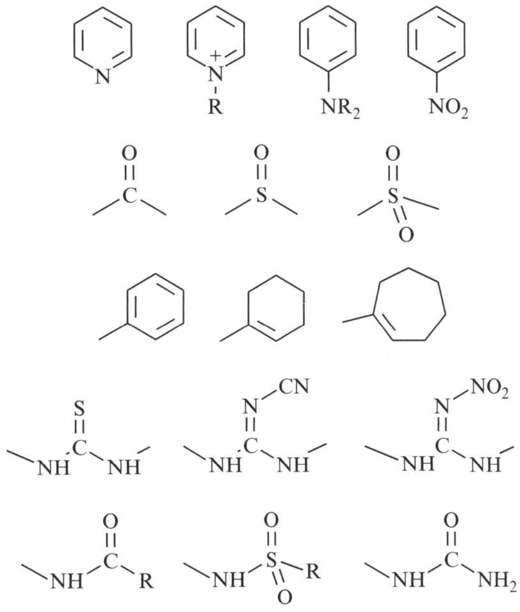

in their chemical and/or physical properties (Table 4.3). As a result, they may exhibit similar pharmacokinetic and pharmacodynamic properties. In other words, the replacement of a substituent by its isostere is more likely to result in the formation of an analogue with the same type of activity as the lead than the totally random selection of an alternative substituent. However, luck still plays a part, and an isosteric analogue may have a totally different type of activity from its lead (see section 2.3 and Figure 4.4).

A large number of drugs have been discovered by isosteric interchanges (Figure 4.4).

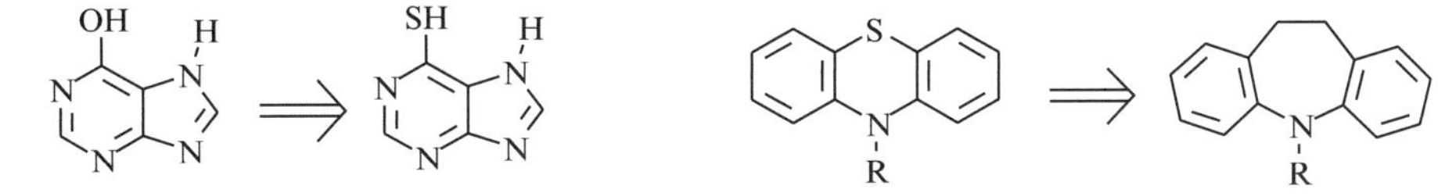

| Hypoxanthine | 6-Mercaptopurine (Antitumour agent) | Phenothiazine drugs (Neuroleptics) | Dibenzazepine drugs (Neuroleptics) |

Figure 4.4 Examples of drugs discovered by isosteric replacement

4.4   Quantitative structure–activity relationships (QSARS)

QSAR is an attempt to remove the element of luck from drug design by establishing a mathematical relationship in the form of an equation between biological activity and measurable physicochemical parameters. These parameters are used to **represent** properties such as lipophilicity, shape and electron distribution, which are believed to have a major influence on the drug's activity. They are normally defined so that they are in the form of numbers, which are derived from practical data that is thought to be related to the property the parameter represents. This makes it possible to either to measure or to calculate these parameters for a group of compounds and relate their values to the biological activity of these compounds by means of mathematical equations using statistical methods such as regression analysis (see Appendix 6). These equations may be used by the medicinal chemist to make a more informed choice as to which analogues to prepare. For example, it is often possible to use statistical data from other compounds to calculate the theoretical value of a specific parameter for an as yet unsynthesized compound. Substituting this value in the appropriate equation relating activity to that parameter, it is possible to calculate the theoretical activity of this unknown compound. Alternatively, the equation could be used to determine the value 'x' of the parameter 'y' that would give optimum activity. As a result, only analogues that have values of y in the region of x need be synthesized.

The main properties of a drug that appear to influence its activity are its, lipophilicity, the electronic effects within the molecule and the size and shape of the molecule (steric effects). Lipophilicity is a measure of a drug's solubility in lipid membranes. This is usually an important factor in determining how easily a drug passes through lipid membranes (see Appendix 5). The electronic effects of the groups within the molecule will affect its electron distribution, which in turn has a direct bearing on how easily and permanently the molecule binds to its target molecule (see Chapter 7). Drug size and shape will determine whether the drug molecule is able to get close enought to its target site in order to bind to that site. The parameters commonly used to represent these properties are partition coefficients for lipohilicity (see section 4.4.1), Hammett σ constants for electronic effects (see section 4.4.2) and Taft M_s steric constants for steric effects (see section 4.4.3). Consequently, this text will be largely restricted to a discussion of the use of these constants. However, the other parameters mentioned in this and other texts are normally used in a similar fashion.

QSAR derived equations take the general form:

$$\text{biological activity} = \text{function}\{\text{parameter(s)}\} \qquad (4.1)$$

in which the activity is normally expressed as log[1/(concentration term)], usually C, the minimum concentration required to cause a defined biological response. Where there is a poor correlation between the values of a specific parameter and the drug's activity, other parameters must be playing a more important part in the drug's action, and so they must also be incorporated into the QSAR equation.

QSAR studies are normally carried out on groups of related compounds. However, QSAR studies on structurally diverse sets of compounds are becoming more common. In both instances it is important to consider as wide a range of parameters as possible.

4.4.1 Lipophilicity

Two parameters are commonly used to represent lipophilicity, namely the partition coefficient (P) and the lipophilicity substituent constant (π). The former parameter refers to the whole molecule whilst the latter is related to substituent groups.

Partition coefficients (P)

A drug has to pass through a number of biological membranes in order to reach its site of action. Consequently, organic medium/aqueous system partition coefficients were the obvious parameters to use as a measure of the ease of movement of the drug through these membranes. The accuracy of the correlation of drug activity with partition coefficients will depend on the solvent system used as a model for the membrane. A variety of organic solvents, such as n-octanol, chloroform and olive oil, are used to represent the membrane (organic medium), whilst both pure water and buffered solutions are used for the aqueous medium. The n-octanol–water system is frequently chosen because it appears to be a good mimic of lipid polarity and has an extensive database. However, more accurate results may be obtained if the organic phase is matched to the area of biological activity being studied. For example, n-octanol usually gives the most consistent results for drugs absorbed in the GI tract whilst less polar solvents such as olive oil frequently give more consistent correlations for drugs crossing the blood–brain barrier. More polar solvents such as chloroform give more consistent values for buccal absorption (soft tissues in the mouth).

The nature of the relationship between P and drug activity depends on the range of P values obtained for the compounds used. If this range is small the results may be expressed as a straight line equation having the general form:

$$\log(1/C) = k_1 \log P + k_2 \tag{4.2}$$

where k_1 and k_2 are constants. This equation indicates a linear relationship between the activity of the drug and its partition coefficient. Over larger ranges of P values the graph of log $1/C$ against log P often has a parabolic form (Figure 4.5) with a maximum value (log P^0). The existence of this maximum value implies that there is an optimum balance between aqueous and lipid solubility for maximum biological activity. Below P^0 the drug will be reluctant to enter the membrane whilst above P^0 the drug will be reluctant to leave the membrane. Log P^0 represents the optimum partition coefficient for biological activity. This means that analogues with partition coefficients near this optimum value are likely to be the most active and worth further investigation. Hansch $et\ al.$ showed that many of these parabolic relationships could be represented reasonably accurately by equations of the form:

$$\log(1/C) = -k_1(\log P)^2 + k_2 \log P + k_3 \tag{4.3}$$

where k_1, k_2 and k_3 are constants that are normally determined by regression analysis.

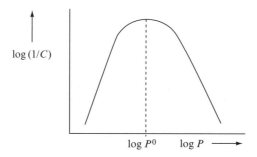

Figure 4.5   A parabolic plot for log $(1/C)$ against log P

Lipophilic substituent constants (π)

Lipophilic substituent constants are also known as hydrophobic substituent constants. They represent the contribution that a group makes to the partition coefficient and were defined by Hansch and co-workers by the equation:

$$\pi = \log P_{RH} - \log P_{RX} \tag{4.4}$$

where P_{RH} and P_{RX} are the partition coefficients of the standard compound and its monosubstituted derivative respectively. However, when several substituents are present, the value of π for the compound is the sum of the π values of each of the separate substituents.

The value of π for a specific substituent will vary with the structural environment of the substituent (Table 4.4). Consequently, average values or the values relevant to the type of structure being investigated may be used in determining activity relationships. It also depends on the solvent system used to determine the partition coefficients. The values of π will also depend on the solvent system used to determine the partition coefficients used in their calculation. Most values are determined using the n-octanol/water system. A positive π value indicates that a substituent has a higher lipophilicity than hydrogen and so will probably increase the concentration of the compound in the n-octanol layer and by inference its concentration in the lipid material of biological systems. Conversely, a negative π value shows that the substituent has a lower lipophilicity than hydrogen and so probably increases the concentration of the compound in the aqueous media of biological systems. Furthermore, biological activity–π relationships that have high regression constants (Appendix 6) and low standard deviations demonstrate that the substituents are important in determining the lipophilic character of the drug.

Table 4.4 Examples of the variations of π values with chemical structure

Substituent X	Aliphatic systems R–X	⟨⟩–X	O_2N–⟨⟩–X	HO–⟨⟩–X
–H	0.00	0.00	0.00	0.00
–CH₃	0.50	0.56	0.52	0.49
–F	−0.17	0.14		0.31
–Cl	0.39	0.71	0.54	0.93
–OH	−1.16	−0.67	0.11	−0.87
–NH₂		−1.23	−0.46	−1.63
–NO₂		−0.28	−0.39	0.50
–OCH₃	0.47	−0.02	0.18	−0.12

Lipophilic constants are frequently used when dealing with a series of analogues in which only the substituents are different. This usage is based on the assumption that the lipophilic effect of the unchanged part of the structure is similar for each of the analogues.

4.4.2 Electronic effects

The distribution of the electrons in a drug molecule has a considerable influence on the distribution and activity of a drug. In general, nonpolar and polar drugs in their unionized form are more readily transported through membranes than polar drugs and drugs in their ionized forms. Furthermore, once the drug reaches its target site the distribution of electrons in its structure will control the type of bond it forms with that target, which in turn affects its biological activity. The first attempt to quantify the electronic affects of groups on the physicochemical properties of compounds was made by Hammett (ca. 1940).

4.4.2.1 The Hammett constant (σ)

The distribution of electrons within a molecule depends on the nature of the electron withdrawing and donating groups found in that structure. Hammett used this concept to calculate what are now known as **Hammett constants (σ_X)** for a variety of monosubstituted benzoic acids (Equation (4.5)). He used these constants to calculate equilibrium and rate constants for chemical reactions. However, they are now used as electronic parameters in QSAR relationships. Hammett constants (σ_X) are defined as:

$$\sigma_X = \log(K_{BX}/K_B) \tag{4.5}$$

that is

$$\sigma_X = \log K_{BX} - \log K_B \tag{4.6}$$

and so, as $pK_a = -\log K_a$,

$$\sigma_X = pK_B - pK_{BX} \tag{4.7}$$

where K_B and K_{BX} are the equilibrium constants for benzoic acid and mono-substituted benzoic acids respectively. Its value varies depending on whether the substituent is an overall electron donor or acceptor. A negative value for σ_X indicates that the substituent is acting as an electron donor group since $K_B > K_{BX}$. Conversely, a positive value for σ_X shows that the substituent is acting as an electron withdrawing group as $K_B < K_{BX}$. The value of σ_X for a specific substituent contains both inductive and mesomeric (resonance) contributions, and so varies with the position of that substituent in the molecule. This variation is indicated by the use of the subscripts m and p (Table 4.5). Inductive and Swain–Lupton constants are attempts to quantify the inductive and mesomeric effects of a substituent.

Table 4.5 Examples of the different electronic substitution constants used in QSAR studies. Inductive substituent constants (σ_1) are the contribution the inductive effect makes to Hammett constants and can be used for aliphatic compounds. Taft substitution constants (σ^*) refer to aliphatic substituents but use propanoic acid (the 2-methyl derivative of ethanoic acid) as the reference point. The Swain–Lupton constants represent the contributions due to the inductive (F) and mesomeric or resonance (R) components of Hammett constants. Adapted from *An Introduction to the Principles of Drug Design and Action* by Smith and Williams 3rd Ed. (1998) Ed. H.J.Smith. Reproduced by permission of Harwood Academic Publishers.

Substituent	Hammett constants		Inductive constants	Taft constants	Swain–Lupton constants	
	σ_m	σ_p	σ_1	σ^*	F	R
–H	0.00	0.00	0.00	0.49	0.00	0.00
–CH$_3$	−0.07	−0.17	−0.05	0.00	−0.04	−0.13
–C$_2$H$_5$	−0.07	−0.15	−0.05	−0.10	−0.05	−0.10
–Ph	0.06	−0.01	0.10	0.60	0.08	−0.08
–OH	0.12	−0.37	0.25	—	0.29	−0.64
–Cl	0.37	0.23	0.47	—	0.41	−0.15
–NO$_2$	0.71	0.78	—	—	0.67	0.16

Hammett postulated that the σ values calculated for the ring substituents of a series of benzoic acids could also be valid for those ring substituents in a different series of similar aromatic compounds. This relationship has been found to be in good agreement for the meta and para substituents of a wide variety of aromatic compounds but not for their ortho substituents. The latter is believed to be due to steric hindrance and other effects, such as intramolecular hydrogen bonding.

Hammett substitution constants suffer from the disadvantage that they only apply to substituents directly attached to a benzene ring. Consequently, a number of other electronic constants (Table 4.5) have been introduced and used in QSAR studies in a similar manner to the Hammett constants. However, attempts to relate biological activity exclusively to the values of Hammett substitution and similar constants have been largely unsuccessful, since electron distribution is not the only factor involved (see section 4.4).

4.4.3 Steric effects

The first parameter used to show the relationship between the shape and size (bulk) of a drug, the dimensions of its target site and the drug's activity was the Taft steric parameter (E_s). It was followed by Charton's steric parameter (v), Verloop's steric parameters and the molar refractivity (MR) amongst others. The most used of these additional parameters is probably the molar refractivity.

4.4.3.1 The Taft steric parameter (E_s)

Taft (1956) used the relative rate constants of the acid catalysed hydrolysis of α-substituted methyl ethanoates to define his steric parameter because it had been shown that the rates of these hydrolyses were almost entirely dependent on steric factors. He used methyl ethanoate as his standard and defined E_s as:

$$E_s = \log\frac{k_{(XCH_2COOCH_3)}}{k_{(CH_3COOCH_3)}} = \log k_{(XCH_2COOCH_3)} - \log k_{(CH_3COOCH_3)} \qquad (4.8)$$

where k is the rate constant of the appropriate hydrolysis and the value of $E_s = 0$ when X $=$ CH_3. It is assumed that the values for E_s (Table 4.6.) obtained for a group using the hydrolysis data are applicable to other structures containing that group. The methyl based E_s values can be converted to H based values by adding -1.24 to the corresponding methyl based values.

Table 4.6 Examples of the Taft steric parameter E_s

Group	E_s	Group	E_s	Group	E_s
H–	1.24	F–	0.78	CH_3O–	0.69
CH_3–	0.00	Cl–	0.27	CH_3S–	0.19
C_2H_5–	−0.07	F_3C–	−1.16	$PhCH_2$–	−0.38
$(CH_3)_2$ CH–	−0.47	Cl_3C–	−2.06	PhOCH–	−0.33

Taft steric parameters have been found to be useful in a number of investigations (see section 4.4.4). They also suffer from the disadvantage that they are determined by experiment. This has limited the number of values recorded in the literature.

4.4.3.2 Molar refractivity (MR)

The molar refractivity is a measure of both the volume of a compound and how easily it is polarized. It is defined as:

$$MR = \frac{(n^2 - 1)M}{(n^2 + 2)\rho} \qquad (4.9)$$

where n is the refractive index, M the relative mass and ρ the density of the compound. The M/ρ term is a measure of the molar volume whilst the refractive index term is a measure of the polarizability of the compound. Although MR is calculated for the whole molecule, it is an additive parameter, and so the MR values for a molecule can be calculated by adding together the MR values for its component parts (Table 4.7).

Table 4.7 Examples of calculated MR values. Reproduced by permission of John Wiley and Sons Ltd. from Hansch C. and Leo A.J. *Substituents Constants for Correlation Analysis in Chemistry and Biology* (1979)

Group	MR	Group	MR	Group	MR
H–	1.03	F–	0.92	CH_3O–	7.87
CH_3–	5.65	Cl–	6.03	HO–	2.85
C_2H_5–	10.30	F_3C–	5.02	CH_3CONH–	14.93
$(CH_3)_2CH$–	14.96	O_2N–	7.63	CH_3CO–	11.18

4.4.3.3 Other parameters

These can be broadly divided into those that apply to sections of the molecule and those that involve the whole molecule. The former include parameters such as van der Waals' radii, Charton's steric constants and the Verloop steric parameters. The latter range from relative molecular mass (RMM) and molar volumes to surface area. They have all been used to correlate biological activity to structure with varying degrees of success.

4.4.4 Hansch analysis

Hansch analysis attempts to mathematically relate drug activity to measurable chemical properties. It is based on Hansch's proposal that drug action could be divided into two stages:

1. the transport of the drug to its site of action;

2. the binding of the drug to the target site.

Each of these stages is dependent on the chemical and physical properties of the drug and its target site. In Hansch analysis these properties are described by the parameters discussed in sections 4.4.1, 4.4.2 and 4.4.3 as well as other parameters. Hansch postulated that the biological activity of a drug could be related to these parameters by simple mathematical relationships based on the general format:

$$\log 1/C = k_1(\text{partition parameter}) + k_2(\text{electronic parameter}) + k_3(\text{steric parameter}) + k_4 \quad (4.10)$$

where C is the minimum concentration required to cause a specific biological response and k_1, k_2, k_3 and k_4 are numerical constants obtained by feeding the values of the parameters selected by the investigating team into a suitable computer statistical package. These parameter values are obtained either from the literature (e.g. π, σ and E_s) or determined by experiment (e.g. C, P etc.). In investigations where more than one substituent is changed, the value of a specific parameter may be expressed in the Hansch equation as either the sum of the values of that parameter for the individual substituents or independent individual parameters. For example, in the hypothetical case of a benzene ring with two substituents X and Y the Hammett constants could be expressed in the Hansch equation as either $k_1 \sum(\sigma_X + \sigma_Y)$ or $k_1\sigma_X + k_2\sigma_Y$. The equations obtained from the selected data are commonly referred to as **Hansch equations**. Their precise nature varies (Table 4.8), but for an investigation using P, σ and E_s Hansch equations often takes the general form:

$$\log 1/C = k_1 P - k_2 P^2 + k_3\sigma + k_4 E_S + k_5 \quad (4.11)$$

Parameters other than those shown in equation (4.11) may be used to derive Hansch equations. A comprehensive list may be found in a review by Tute in *Advances in Drug Research* 1971, **6**, 1.

The accuracy of a Hansch equation will depend on:

1. the number of analogues (n) used: the greater the number the higher the probability of obtaining an accurate Hansch equation;

2. the accuracy of the biological data used in the derivation of the equation. The degree of variation normally found in biological measurements means that a statistically viable number of measurements should be taken for each analogue and an average value used in the derivation of the Hansch equation;

3. the choice of parameter (see 'Craig plots' below).

Table 4.8 Examples of simple Hansch equations

Compound	Activity	Hansch equation
	Antiadrenergic	$\log 1/C = 1.22\pi - 1.59\sigma + 7.89$ $(n = 22; s = 0.238; r = 0.918)$
	Antibiotic (*in vivo*)	$\log 1/C = -0.445\pi + 5.673$ $(n = 20; r = 0.909)$
	MAO inhibitor (humans)	$\log 1/C = 0.398\pi + 1.089\sigma + 1.03E_s + 4.541$ $(n = 9; r = 0.955))$
	Concentration (C_b) in the brain after 15 minutes	$\log C_b = 0.765\pi - 0.540\pi^2 + 1.505$

The accuracy of a Hansch equation may be assessed from the values of the standard deviation (*s*) and the regression constant (*r*) given by the statistical package used to obtain the equation. The smaller the value of *s* the better the data fits the equation. Values of *r* that are significantly lower than 0.9 indicate that either unsuitable parameter(s) were used to derive the equation or there is no relationship between the compounds used and their activity. This suggests that the mechanisms by which these compounds act are unrelated because the mechanisms are very different from each other.

Hansch equations may be used to predict the activity of an as yet unsynthesized analogue. This enables the medicinal chemist to make an informed choice as to which analogues are worth synthesizing. However, these predictions should only be regarded as valid if they are made within the range of parameter values used to establish the Hansch equation. Furthermore, when the predicted activity is widely different from the observed value, it indicates that the activity is affected by factors, such as the ease of metabolism, that were not included in the derivation of the Hansch equation.

Hansch analysis may also be used to give an indication of the importance of the influence of a parameter on the mechanism by which a drug acts. Consider, for example, a series of analogues whose activity is related to the parameters π and σ by the hypothetical Hansch equation:

$$\log 1/C = 1.78\pi - 0.12\sigma + 1.674 \qquad (4.12)$$

The small value of the coefficient for σ relative to that of π in equation (4.12) shows that the electronic effects do not play an important part in the action of the drug.

Craig plots

Craig plots are two dimensional plots of one parameter against another (Figure 4.6). The plot is divided into four sections corresponding to the positive and negative values of the parameters. They are used, in conjunction with an already established Hansch equation for a series of related aromatic compounds, to select the aromatic substituents that are likely to produce highly active

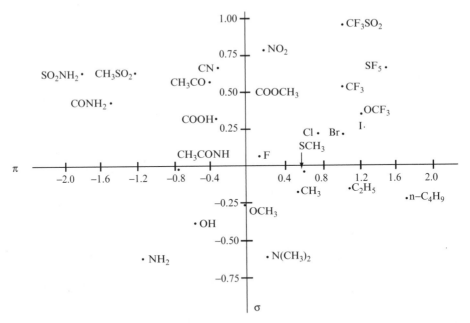

Figure 4.6 An example of a Craig plot of para Hammett constants σ against para π values. [Reprinted with permission of John Wiley and Sons, Inc. from Craig P N (1980). In *Burgers Medicinal Chemistry* (M E Wolff, Ed.) 4th ed., Part 1 p. 343. Wiley, New York. Copyright © [1980 John Wiley and Sons Inc.]

analogues. For example, suppose that a Hansch analysis carried out on a series of aromatic compounds yields the Hansch equation:

$$\log 1/C = 2.67\pi - 2.56\sigma + 3.92 \qquad (4.13)$$

To obtain a high value for the activity (1/C) it is necessary to pick substituents with a positive π value and a negative σ value. In other words, if high activity analogues are required, the substituents should be chosen from the lower right-hand quadrant of the plot. However, it is emphasized that the use of a Craig plot does not guarantee that the resultant analogues will be more active than the lead because the parameters used may not be relevant to the mechanism by which the analogue acts.

4.5   The Topliss decision tree

The Topliss decision tree is essentially a flow diagram that in a series of steps directs the medicinal chemist to produce a series of analogues, some of which should have a greater activity than the lead used to start the tree. It is emphasized that only some of the compounds will be more active than the lead compound. The method is most useful when it is not possible to make the large number of compounds necessary to produce an accurate Hansch equation. However, its use is limited because it requires the lead compound to have an unfused aromatic ring system and it only produces analogues that are substituents of that aromatic system. In addition, the Topliss method also depends on the user being able to rapidly measure the biological activity of the lead compound and its analogues.

There are two Topliss decision trees (Figure 4.7), one for substituents directly attached to an aromatic ring and the other for changes in the aliphatic side chains of an aromatic ring system. Both are used in a similar manner. In both cases the investigation starts with the conversion of the lead into the first analogue at the top of the tree, either the 4-chloro analogue (Figure 4.7(a)) or the isopropyl analogue (Figure 4.7(b)). The activity of this analogue is measured and classified as either less (L), approximately the same (E) or significantly greater (M) than that of the original lead. If the activity is greater than that of the lead the next analogue to be prepared is the next one on the M route. Alternatively, if the activity of the analogue is less than that of the original lead the next step is to produce the analogue indicated by the L route on the tree. Similarly, if the activity is about the same as that of the original lead the E route

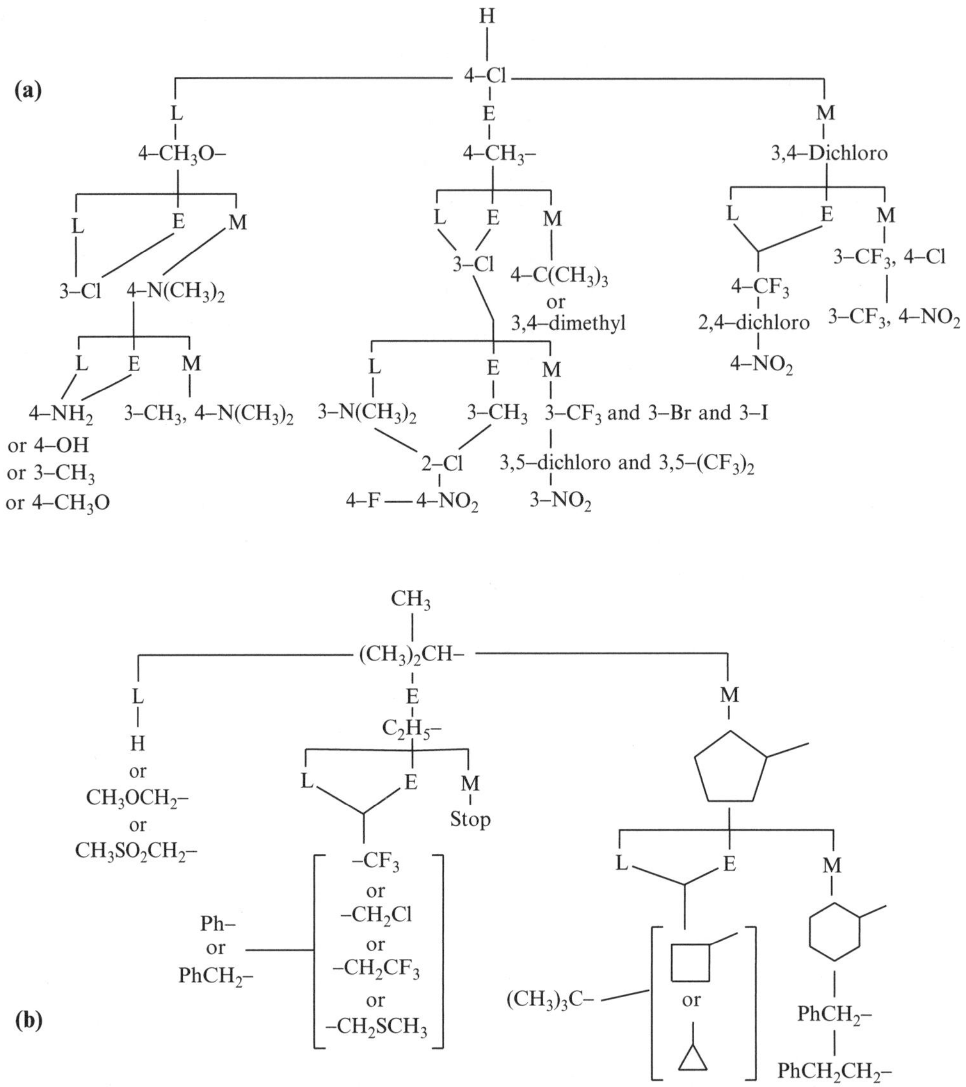

(a)

H
|
4–Cl

L — E — M

L: 4–CH$_3$O–

L — E — M

3–Cl   4–N(CH$_3$)$_2$

L — E — M

4–NH$_2$
or 4–OH
or 3–CH$_3$
or 4–CH$_3$O

3–CH$_3$, 4–N(CH$_3$)$_2$

E: 4–CH$_3$–

L — E — M

3–Cl   4–C(CH$_3$)$_3$
or
3,4–dimethyl

L — E — M

3–N(CH$_3$)$_2$ 3–CH$_3$ 3–CF$_3$ and 3–Br and 3–I

2–Cl   3,5–dichloro and 3,5–(CF$_3$)$_2$

4–F — 4–NO$_2$ 3–NO$_2$

M: 3,4–Dichloro

L — E — M

4–CF$_3$ 3–CF$_3$, 4–Cl

2,4–dichloro   3–CF$_3$, 4–NO$_2$

4–NO$_2$

(b)

CH$_3$
|
(CH$_3$)$_2$CH–

L — E — M

L: H
or
CH$_3$OCH$_2$–
or
CH$_3$SO$_2$CH$_2$–

E: C$_2$H$_5$–

L — E — M

Ph–
or
PhCH$_2$–

–CF$_3$
or
–CH$_2$Cl
or
–CH$_2$CF$_3$
or
–CH$_2$SCH$_3$

Stop

M:

L — E — M

(CH$_3$)$_3$C–   or   ▢ △

PhCH$_2$–

PhCH$_2$CH$_2$–

Figure 4.7 The Topliss decision trees for (a) an unfused aromatic ring and (b) an aliphatic side chain. (L = significantly lower activity, E = about the same activity and M = significantly greater activity). Reproduced by permission of Taylor and Francis Ltd. from the *Journal of Medicinal Chemistry* 15, No. 10 1006 (1972), http://www.tandf.co.uk/journals. Utilisation of Operational Schemes for Analog Synthesis in Drug Design by J G Topliss

is followed and the appropriate analogue synthesized. This procedure is repeated, the activity of each new analogue being compared with that of its precursor in order to determine which branch of the tree gives the next analogue. Suppose, for example, that a compound A (Figure 4.8) is active against

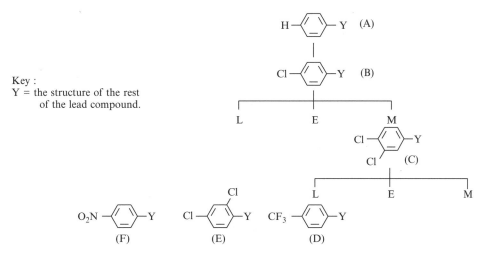

Key :
Y = the structure of the rest
    of the lead compound.

Figure 4.8   A hypothetical example of the use of the Topliss decision tree. The compounds are synthesized in the order A, B, C, ... etc. It should be realized that only some of the compounds synthesized will be more potent than the original lead A

S. aureus and activity of this compound and its analogues can be readily assessed by a biological method. The first step in the Topliss approach is to synthesize the 4-chloro derivative (B) of A. Suppose the activity of B is greater than that of A, then following the M branch the Topliss tree (Figure 4.8) indicates that the next analogue to produce is the 3,4-dichloro derivative (C) of A. Once again suppose that the biological assay of C was less than that of B. In this case, the Topliss tree shows that the next most promising analogue is the 4-trifluromethyl derivative of (D) of A. At this point one would also synthesize and biologically test the 2,4-dichloro (E) and the 4-nitro analogues (F) of A. It is emphasized that the decision tree is not a synthetic pathway for the production of each of the analogues. It simply suggests which of the substituents would be likely to yield a more potent analogue. The synthetic route for producing each of the suggested analogues would vary for each analogue and would use the most appropriate starting materials.

The Topliss decision tree does not give all the possible analogues but it is likely that a number of the most active analogues will be found by this method.

4.6   Questions

(1)   State the full wording of the abbreviation 'SAR'. Describe the general way in which SAR is used to develop a drug. Illustrate the answer by reference to the changes in the activities of 4-alkylresorcinols caused by changes in the chain length of the 4-alkyl group.

(2)   (i) How would the introduction of a chloro group be expected to affect the character of the resulting analogue?
      (ii) What alternative halogen containing group could be used in place of chlorine? Give one reason for the use of this group.

(3)   Explain the meaning of the terms (i) isostere and (ii) bioisostere.

(4)   Suggest how the introduction of each of the following groups into the structure of a lead could be expected to affect the bioavailability of the resultant analogue: (i) a sulphonic acid group, (ii) a methyl group and (iii) a hydroxy group. Assume that these groups are introduced into the section of the lead's structure that does not contain its pharmacophore.

(5)   Outline the fundamental principle underlying the QSAR approach to drug design.

(6)   Lipophilicity, shape and electron distribution all have a major influence on drug activity. State the parameters that are commonly used as a measure of these properties in the QSAR approach to drug design.

(7)   (a) Describe the approach to drug design known as Hansch analysis.
      (b) Phenols are antiseptics. Hansch analysis carried out on a series of phenols with the general structure A yielded the Hansch equation

$$\log 1/C = 1.5\pi - 0.2\sigma + 2.3$$
$$n = 23, \ s = 0.13, \ r = 0.87$$

(A)   R $-\!\!\!\left\langle\!\!\!\begin{array}{c}/\!\!/\ \ \backslash\backslash\\ \underline{\quad}\end{array}\!\!\!\right\rangle\!\!\!-$ OH

What is (i) the significance of the terms n, s and r, (ii) the relative significance of the lipophilicity and electronic distribution of a phenol of type A on its activity and (iii) the effect of replacing the R group of A by a more polar group?

(continued)

(8) (a) How are Craig plots used in Hansch analysis? (b) Use Figure 4.6 to predict
     the structures of the analogues of compond A in question (7) that would
     be likely to have a high antiseptic activity.

(9) (i) Describe how the Topliss decision tree is used in drug design.
     (ii) What are the major limitations to its use?

5 Computer Aided Drug Design

5.1 Introduction

The development of powerful desk top and larger computers has enabled chemists to predict the structures and the values of properties of known, unknown, stable and unstable molecular species using mathematical equations. These equations are obtained using so called 'models' of the system being studied (see sections 5.2 and 5.3). Solving these equations gives the required data. The reliability of the mathematical methods used to obtain and solve the equations is well known and so in most cases it is possible to obtain a reliable estimate of the accuracy of the results. In some cases the calculated values are believed to be more accurate than the experimentally determined figures because of the higher degree of experimental error in the experimental work. Graphics packages that convert the data for the structure of a chemical species into a variety of easy to understand visual formats have also been developed (Figure 5.1). Consequently, in medicinal chemistry, it is now possible to visualize the three dimensional shapes of both the ligands and their target sites. In addition, sophisticated computational chemistry packages also allow the medicinal chemist to evaluate the interactions between a compound and its target site before synthesizing that compound (see section 5.5). This means that the medicinal chemist need only synthesize and test the most promising of the compounds, which considerably increases the chances of discovering a potent drug. It also significantly reduces the cost of development.

Molecular modelling is a complex subject and it is not possible to cover it in depth in this text. For workers wishing to use it as a tool in drug design it will be necessary to either ask a competent **computational chemist** to make the necessary calculations and graphic conversions or to treat the computer as a **black box** and use the relevant computer program according to its manufacturer's instructions. In both approaches to molecular modelling, it is essential that the drug designer

Fundamentals of Medicinal Chemistry, Edited by Gareth Thomas
© 2003 John Wiley & Sons, Ltd
ISBN 0 470 84306 3 (Hbk), ISBN 0 470 84307 1 (pbk)

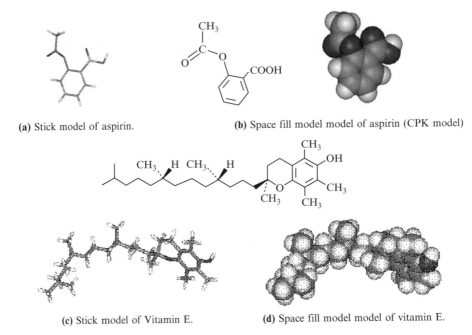

(a) Stick model of aspirin.   **(b)** Space fill model model of aspirin (CPK model)

(c) Stick model of Vitamin E.   **(d)** Space fill model model of vitamin E.

Figure 5.1 Examples of some of the formats used by graphics packages to display molecular models on computer screens

has a basic understanding of the fundamental concepts of the methods used in order to avoid making incorrect deductions, as well as to appreciate the limitations of the methods.

5.1.1 Molecular modelling methods

The three dimensional shapes of both ligand and target site may be determined by X-ray crystallography or computational methods. The most common computational methods are based on either molecular or quantum mechanics. Both these approaches produce equations for the total energy of the structure. In these equations the positions of the atoms in the structure are represented by either Cartesian or polar coordinates (Figure 5.2). In the past, the initial values of these atomic coordinates were set by the modeller. However, as it is now customary to construct models from existing structural fragments (see section 5.2.1) modern computer programs will automatically set up the coordinates of the atoms in the first fragment from the program's database. As additional fragments are added, the the computer automatically adjusts the coordinates of

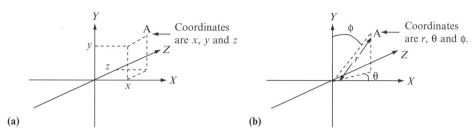

Figure 5.2   (a) Cartesian and (b) polar coordinates of point A

the atoms of these additional fragments to values that are relative to those of the first fragment, since it is the relative positions of the atoms that is important as regards the energy of the structure, and not the absolute positions of the atoms. Once the energy equation is established, the computer computes the set of coordinates which correspond to a minimum total energy value for the system. This set of coordinates is converted into the required visual display by the graphics package (Figure 5.1). However, although the calculations made by computers are always accurate, the calculated result should be checked for accuracy against experimental observations. In this respect it is essential that the approximations on which the calculations are based are understood. For example, most calculations are based on a frozen molecule at 0 K in a vacuum and so do not take into account that the structure is vibrating or the influence of the medium in which the chemical species is found. Calculations taking these factors into account would undoubtedly give a more realistic picture of the structure.

Quantum mechanics calculations are more expensive to carry out because they require considerable more computing power and time than molecular mechanics calculations. Consequently, molecular mechanics is the more useful source of the large structures of interest to the medicinal chemist and so this chapter will concentrate on this method. To save time and expense, structures are often built up using information obtained from databases, such as the Cambridge and Brookhaven databases. Information from databases may also be used to check the accuracy of the modelling technique. However, in all cases, the accuracy of the structures obtained will depend on the accuracy of the data used in their determination. Furthermore, it must be appreciated that the molecular models produced by computers are a caricature of reality that simply provide us with a useful picture for design and communication purposes. It is important to realize that we still do not know what molecules actually look like!

5.1.2 Computer graphics

In molecular modelling the data produced are converted into visual images on a computer screen by graphics packages. These images may be displayed as space fill, CPK (Corey–Pauling–Koltun), stick, ball and stick, mesh and ribbon (see Figure 5.1 and Figure 5.3(a), 5.3(b) and 5.3(c)). Ribbon representations are usually used to depict large molecules, such as nucleic acids and proteins. Each of these formats can, if required, use a colour code to represent the different elements, for example, carbon atoms are usually green, oxygen red and nitrogen blue. However, most graphics packages will allow the user to change this code. The program usually indicates the three dimensional nature of the molecule by making the colours of the structure lighter the further it is from the viewer. Structures may be displayed in their minimum energy or other energy states. They may be shrunk or expanded to a desired size as well as rotated about either the x or y axis. These facilities enable the molecule to be viewed from different angles and also allows the structure to be fitted to its target site (see section 5.5). In addition, it is possible using molecular dynamics (see section 5.4) to show how the shape of the structure might vary with time by visualizing the natural vibrations of the molecule (Figure 5.3(d)) as a moving image on the screen. However, it is emphasized that both the stationary and moving images shown on the screen are useful caricatures and not pictures of the real structure of the molecule.

5.2   Molecular mechanics

Molecular mechanics is the more popular of the methods used to obtain molecular models as it is simpler to use and requires considerably less computing time to produce a model. The molecular mechanics method is based on the assumption that the relative positions of the nuclei of the atoms forming a structure are determined by the forces of attraction and repulsion operating in that structure. It assumes that the total **potential energy** (E_{Total}) of a molecule is given by the sum of all the energies of the attractive and repulsive forces between the atoms in the structure. These energies are calculated using a mechanical model in which these atoms are represented by balls whose mass is proportional to their relative atomic masses joined by mechanical springs corresponding to the covalent bonds in the structure. Using this model, E_{Total} may be expressed mathematically by equations, known as **force fields**. These equations normally take the general form:

$$E_{Total} = \Sigma E_{Stretching} + \Sigma E_{Bend} + \Sigma E_{Torsion} + \Sigma E_{vdW} \ \Sigma E_{Coulombic} \qquad (5.1)$$

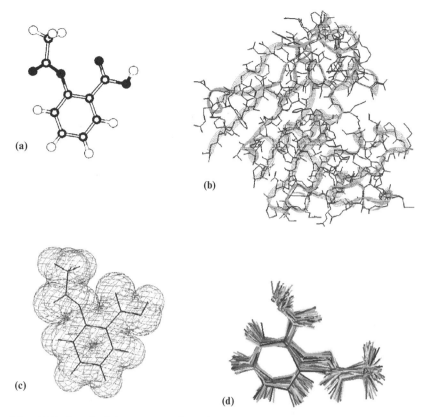

Figure 5.3 (a) Ball and stick representation of aspirin. (b) Ribbon representation of dihydrofo-late reductase. (c) Mesh representation of aspirin. This representation shown simultaneously both the space fill and stick structures of the molecule. (d) Molecular dynamics representation of aspirin at 500 K. The relative movement of the atoms with time within the molecule is indicated by the use of multiple lines between the atoms

where $E_{Stretching}$ is the bond stretching energy (Figure 5.4), E_{Bend} is the bond energy due to changes in bonding angle (Table 5.1), $E_{Torsion}$ is the bond energy due to changes in the conformation of a bond (Table 5.1), E_{vdW} is the total energy contribution due to van der Waals forces and $E_{Coulombic}$ the electrostatic attractive and repulsive forces operating in the molecule between atoms carrying a partial or full charge. Other energy terms, such as one for hydrogen bonding, may be added as required. Each of these energy terms includes expressions for all the specified interactions between all the atoms in the molecule.

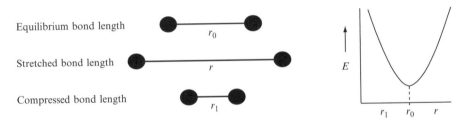

Figure 5.4 Bond stretching and compression related to the changes in the potential energy (E) of the system

The values of each of the energy terms in Equation (5.1) are calculated by considering the mechanical or electrical nature of the structure that the energy term represents. For example, the $E_{\text{Stretching}}$ bond stretching energy for a pair of atoms joined by a single covalent bond may be estimated by considering the bond to be a mechanical spring that obeys **Hooke's law**. If r is the stretched length of the bond and r_0 is the ideal bond length, that is the length the bond wants to be, then:

$$E_{\text{Streching}} = \tfrac{1}{2}k(r - r_0)^2 \tag{5.2}$$

where k is the force constant, which may be thought of as being a measure of the strength of the spring, in other words a measure of the strength of a bond. For example, C–C bonds have a smaller k value than C$=$C bonds, that is C$=$C bonds are stronger than C–C bonds. In reality, more complex mathematical expressions, such as those given by the Morse function, would probably be used to describe bond stretching.

The value of $\Sigma E_{\text{Stretching}}$ in the force field equation (see equation (5.1)) for a structure is given by the sum of appropriate expressions for E for every pair of bonded atoms in the structure. For example, using the Hooke law model, for a molecule consisting of three atoms bonded a–b–c the expression would be:

$$\Sigma E_{\text{Stretching}} = E_{\text{a-b}} + E_{\text{b-c}} \tag{5.3}$$

that is, the expression for $\Sigma E_{\text{Stretching}}$ in the force field for the molecule would be:

$$\Sigma E_{\text{Stretching}} = \tfrac{1}{2}k_{(a-b)}(r_{(a-b)} - r_{0(a-b)})^2 + \tfrac{1}{2}k_{(b-c)}(r_{(b-c)} - r_{0(b-c)})^2 \tag{5.4}$$

The other energy terms in the force field equation for a structure are treated in a similar manner using expressions appropriate to the mechanical or electrical

Table 5.1 Some of the expressions commonly used to calculate the energy terms given in equation (5.1)

Term	Expression	Model for
E_{Bend}	$E_{Bend} = \frac{1}{2}k_\theta(\theta - \theta_0)^2$ where θ_0 is the ideal bond angle, that is, the minimum energy positions of the three atoms.	*Bond bending*
$E_{Torsion}$	$E_{Torsion} = \frac{1}{2}k_\phi(1 + \cos(m(\phi + \phi_{offset})))$ where k_ϕ is the energy barrier to rotation about the torsion angle ϕ, m is the periodicity of the rotation and ϕ_{offset} is the ideal torsion angle relative (minimum energy positions for the atoms) to a staggered arrangement of the two atoms.	*Rotation about a single bond*
E_{vdW}	$E_{vdW} = \varepsilon[\frac{(r_{min})^{12}}{r} - 2(\frac{r_{min}}{r})^6]$ where r_{min} is the distance between two atoms i and j when the energy is at a minimum ε and r is the actual distance between the atoms. This equation is known as the Lennard-Jones 6–12 potential. The $(\ )^6$ term in this equation represents attractive forces, whilst the $(\ )^{12}$ term represents short range repulsive forces between the atoms.	*Van der Waals non-bonded interactions*
$E_{Coulombic}$	$E_{Coulombic} = \frac{q_i q_j}{D r_{ij}}$ where q_i and q_j are the point charges on atoms i and j, r_{ij} is the distance between the charges and D is the dielectric constant of the medium surrounding the charges.	*Electrostatic coulombic interactions*

model on which the energy term is based (Table 5.1). These expressions may be the equations given in Table 5.1 but, depending on the nature of the system beng modelled, other equations may be a more appropriate way of mathematically describing the mechanical or electrical model.

The values of the parameters r, r_0, k, ... etc used in the expressions for the energy terms in Equation (5.1) are either obtained/calculated from experimental observations or calculated using quantum mechanics using best fit methods. Experimental calculations are based on a wide variety of spectroscopic techniques, thermodynamic data measurements and crystal structure measurements for interatomic distances. Unfortunately, values are often difficult to obtain since accurate experimental data are not always available. Quantum mechanical calculations can be used when experimental information is not available but are expensive on computer time. However, this method does give better values for structures that are not in the minimum energy state. The best fit values are obtained by looking at related structures with known parameter values and using the values from the parts of these structures that most resemble the structure being modelled. Parameter values are also stored in the data bases of the molecular modelling computer programs.

5.2.1 Creating a molecular model using molecular mechanics

Molecular models are usually created by either using an existing commercial force field computer program or assembling a model from structural fragments held in the database of a molecular modelling program. In the former case commercial packages usually have several different force fields within the same package and it is necesary to pick the most appropriate one for the structure being modelled. To use the commercial force field, the values of the relevant parameters together with the initial atomic coordinates are fed into the force field equation. These values are used by the computer to calculate an initial value of E_{Total} for the model. This initial energy value is minimized by the computer iteratively (consecutive repetitive calculations), changing the values of the atomic coordinates in the equation for the force field until a minimum energy value is obtained. The values of the atomic coordinates corresponding to this minimum energy value are used to visualize the model on the monitor screen in an appropriate format (see Figure 5.1 and Figure 5.3(a)–(c)).

The second method assembles the initial model from models of structural fragments held in the database of a molecular modelling program (Figure 5.5). Initially these fragments are put together in a reasonably sensible manner to give a structure that does not allow for steric hindrance. At this point it is necessary to check that the computer has selected atoms for the structure whose configurations correspond to the types of bonding required in the structure, in other words, if an atom is double bonded in the structure, the computer has selected a form of the atom that is double bonded. These checks are carried out by matching a code for the atoms on the screen against the code given in the manual for the program and replacing atoms where necessary. At this stage the structure displayed is not necessarily in its minimum potential energy conformation. However, the program can be instructed to iteratively change the

Step 1: the selection of the structure fragments from the database of the INSIGHT II program. The molecule with the relevant functional group and/or structure is selected.

The INSIGHT II models of these structures.

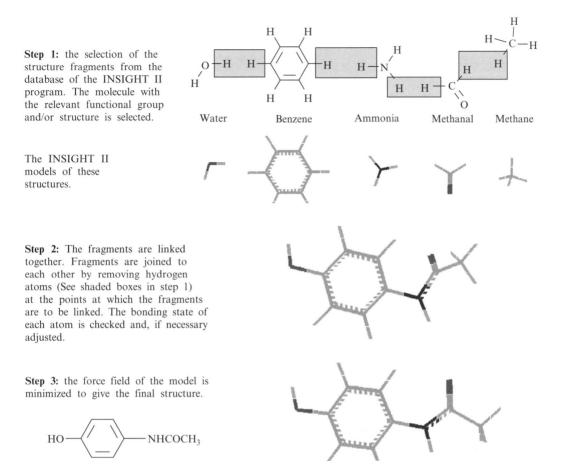

Step 2: The fragments are linked together. Fragments are joined to each other by removing hydrogen atoms (See shaded boxes in step 1) at the points at which the fragments are to be linked. The bonding state of each atom is checked and, if necessary adjusted.

Step 3: the force field of the model is minimized to give the final structure.

HO—⟨ ⟩—NHCOCH$_3$

Figure 5.5 An outline of the steps involved using INSIGHT II to produce a stick model of the structure of paracetamol

atomic coordinates of the model to give a minimum value for E_{Total}. As a result of this change, the structure on the monitor screen assumes a conformation corresponding to a minimum energy state. This conformation may be presented in a number of formats depending on the requirements of the modeller (see Figure 5.1 and Figure 5.3(a)–(c)).

The energy minimizing procedure also automatically twists the molecule to allow for steric hindrance. However, the energy minimizing process is not usually very sophisticated. It stops when the force field reaches the nearest local minimum energy value even though this value is not necessarily the lowest minimum energy value for the structure (Figure 5.6).

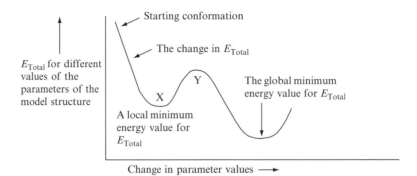

Figure 5.6 A representation of the change in the value of E_{Total} demonstrating how the computation could stop at a local (X) rather than the true (global) minimum value. The use of molecular dynamics gives the structure kinetic energy which allows it to overcome energy barriers, such as Y, to reach the global minimum energy structure of the molecule

Consequently, it may be necessary to use a more sophisticated computer procedure, **molecular dynamics** (section 5.3), to obtain the lowest minimum energy value and as a result the best model for the molecule. This final structure may be moved around the screen and expanded or reduced in size. It can also be rotated about the x or y axis to view different elevations of the molecule.

The molecular mechanics method requires considerably less computing time than the quantum mechanical approach and may be used for large molecules containing more than a thousand atoms. This means that it may be used to model target sites as well as drug and analogue molecules. As well as being used to produce molecular models, it may also be used to provide information about the binding of molecules to receptors (see section 5.5) and the conformational changes (see section 5.3) that occur in the molecule. However, molecular mechanics is not so useful for computing properties, such as electron density, that are related to the electron cloud. Furthermore, it is important to realize that accuracy of the structure obtained will depend on the quality and appropriateness of the parameters used in the force field. Moreover, molecular mechanical calculations are normally based on isolated structures at 0 K and do not normally take into account the effect of the environment on the structure.

5.3 Molecular dynamics

Molecular mechanics calculations are made at 0 K, that is on structures that are frozen in time and so do not show the natural motion of the atoms in those structures. Molecular dynamics programs allow the modeller to show the dynamic nature of molecules by simulating the natural motion of the atoms in a structure. This motion, which is time and temperature dependent, is modelled by including terms for the **kinetic energy** of the atoms in the structure in the force field by using equations based on Newton's laws of motion. The solution of the these force field equations gives coordinates that show how the positions of the atoms in the structure vary with time. These variations are displayed on the monitor in as a moving picture. The appearance of the this picture will depend on the force field selected for the structure and the temperature and time interval used for the integration of the Newtonian equations. Molecular dynamics can also be used to find minimum energy structures (Figure 5.6) and conformational analysis.

5.3.1 Conformational analysis

Each frame of the molecular dynamics 'movie' corresponds to a conformation of the molecule, which may be displayed on the monitor screen in any of the set formats. The program is also able to compute the total energy of each of these conformations and plot a graph of energy against time or degree of rotation (Figure 5.7(a) and (b)). However, this can take some considerable time. For example, it can take several hours of computing time to find all the conformations of a simple molecule containing six bonds if energy calculations are made at a rate of 10 determinations per second.

5.4 Quantum mechanics

Unlike molecular mechanics, the quantum mechanical approach to molecular modelling does not require the use of parameters similar to those used in molecular mechanics. It is based on the realization that electrons and all material particles exhibit wavelike properties. This allows the well defined, parameter free, mathematics of wave motions to be applied to electrons, atomic and molecular structure. The basis of these calculations is the Schrodinger wave equation, which in its simplest form may be stated as:

$$H\Psi = E\Psi \tag{5.5}$$

where Ψ is a mathematical function known as the state function or time-dependent wave function, which defines the state (nature and properties) of a

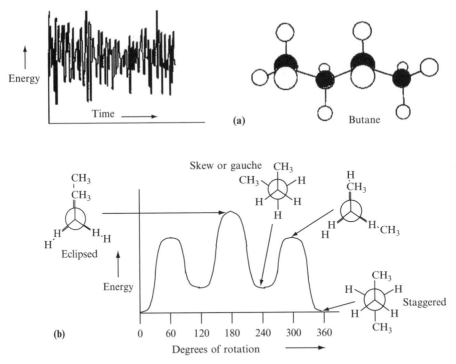

Figure 5.7 (a) Molecular dynamics trajectory for the rotation of the C_2–C_3 bond in butane at 600° using the CAChe program. Moving the cursor along the energy trajectory causes the structure of butane on the right to assume the corresponding conformation. Reproduced from W. B. Smith, *Introduction to Theoretical Organic Chemistry and Molecular Modelling*, 1996, by permission of Wiley–VCH, Inc. (b) A plot of the change in energy with rotation about the C_2–C_3 bond in butane showing the corresponding conformations

system. In molecular modelling terms $E\Psi$ represents the total potential and kinetic energy of all the particles (nuclei and electrons) in the structure and H is the Hamiltonium operator acting on the wave function Ψ. Operators are mathematical methods of converting one function into another function in order to find a solution or solutions of the original function. For example, differentiation is an operator that transforms an equation representing a function into its first derivative.

Schrodinger equations for atoms and molecules use the the sum of the potential and kinetic energies of the electrons and nuclei in a structure as the basis of a description of the three dimensional arangements of electrons about the nucleus. Equations are normally obtained using the Born–Oppenheimer approximation, which considers the nucleus to be stationary with respect to the electrons. This approximation means that one need not consider the kinetic energy of the nuclei in a molecule, which considerably simplifies the calculations. Furthermore, the form of the Schrodinger equations shown in Equation (5.5) is deceptive in that it is not a single equation but represents a set of differential wave equations (Ψ_n), each corresponding to an allowed energy level (E_n) in the structure. The fact that a structure will only possess energy levels with certain specific values is a direct consequence of spectroscopic observations.

The precise mathematical form of $E\,\Psi$ for the Schrodinger equation will depend on the complexity of the structure being modelled. Its operator H will contain individual terms for **all** the possible electron–electron, electron–nucleus and nucleus–nucleus interactions between the electrons and nuclei in the structure needed to determine the energies of the components of that structure. Consider, for example, the structure of the hydrogen molecule with its four particles, namely two electrons at positions r_1 and r_2 and two nuclei at positions R_1 and R_2. The Schrodinger Equation (5.5) may be rewritten for this molecule as:

$$H\Psi = (K + U)\Psi = E\Psi \tag{5.6}$$

where K is the kinetic and U is the potential energy of the two electrons and nuclei forming the structure of the hydrogen molecule. The Hamiltonian operator for this molecule will contain operator terms for all the interactions between these particles and so may be written as:

$$H = -\tfrac{1}{2}\bar{V}_1^2 - \tfrac{1}{2}\bar{V}_2^2 + 1/R_1R_2 - 1/R_1r_1 - 1/R_1r_2 - 1/R_2r_1 - 1/R_2r_2 + 1/r_1r_2 \tag{5.7}$$

where $\tfrac{1}{2}\bar{V}_1^2$ and $\tfrac{1}{2}\bar{V}_2^2$ are terms representing the kinetic energies of the two electrons, and the remaining terms represent all the possible interactions between the relevant electrons and nuclei. The more electrons and nuclei there are in the structure the more complex H becomes and as a direct result the greater the computing time required to obtain solutions of the equation. Consequently, in practice it is not economic to obtain solutions for structures consisting of more than about 50 atoms.

It is not possible to obtain a direct solution of a Schrodinger equation for a structure containing more than two particles. Solutions are normally obtained by simplifying H by using the Hartree–Fock approximation. This approximation uses the concept of an effective field V to represent the interactions of an electron with all the other electrons in the structure. For example, the Hartree–Fock approximation converts the Hamiltonian operator (5.7) for each electron in the hydrogen molecule to the simpler form:

$$H = -\tfrac{1}{2}\bar{V}^2 - 1/R_1r - 1/R_2r + V \qquad (5.8)$$

where r is the position of the electron. The use of the Hartree–Fock approximation reduces computer time and reduces the cost without losing too much in the way of accuracy. Computer time may be further reduced by the use of semi-empirical methods. These methods use experimentally determined data to simplify many of the atomic orbitals, which in turn simplifies the Schrodinger equation for the structure. Solving the Schrodinger equation uses a mathematical method, which is initially based on guessing a solution for each electrons molecular orbital. The computer tests the accuracy of this trial solution and based on its findings modifies the trial solution to produce a new solution. The accuracy of this new solution is tested and a further solution is proposed by the computer. This process is repeated until the testing the solution gives answers within acceptable limits. In molecular modelling the solutions obtained by the use of these methods describe the molecular orbitals of each electron in the molecule. The solutions are normally in the form of sets of equations, which may be interpreted in terms of the probability of finding an electron at specific points in the structure. Graphics programs may be used to convert these probabilities into either presentations like those shown in Figures 5.1 and 5.2 or into electron distribution pictures (Figure 5.8). However, because of the computer time involved, it is not feasible to deal with structures with more than several hundred atoms, which makes the quantum mechanical approach less suitable for large molecules such as the proteins that are of interest to medicinal chemists.

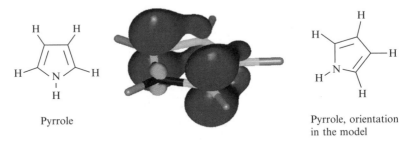

Pyrrole

Pyrrole, orientation
in the model

Figure 5.8 The stick picture of pyrrole on which is superimposed the probability of finding electrons at different points in the molecule obtained using quantum mechanics

Quantum mechanics is useful for calculating the values of ionization potentials, electron affinities, heats of formation and dipole moments and other physical properties of atoms and molecules. It can also be used to calculate the relative probabilities of finding electrons (the electron density) in a structure (Figure 5.8). This makes it possible to determine the most likely points at which a structure will react with electrophiles and nucleophiles. A knowledge of the shape and electron density of a molecule may also be used to assess the nature of the binding of a possible drug to a target site (see section 5.5).

5.5 Docking

The three dimensional structures produced on a computer screen may be manipulated on the screen to show different views of the structures. With more complex molecular mechanics programs it is possible to superimpose one structure on top of another. In other words, it is possible to superimpose the three dimensional structure of a potential drug on its possible target site. This process, which is often automated, is known as **docking** (Figure 5.9). It enables the medicinal chemist to evaluate the fit of potential drugs (ligands) to their target site. If the structure of a ligand is complementary to that of its target site the ligand is more likely to be biologically active. Furthermore, the use of a colour code to indicate the nature of the atoms and functional groups present in the three dimensional structures also enables the medicinal chemist to investigate the binding of the ligand to the target site.

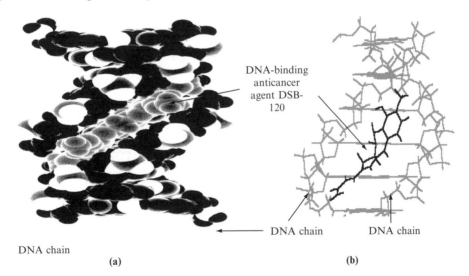

Figure 5.9   The docking of DBS-120 to a fragment of DNA. (a) CPK model; (b) Dreiding model. (Courtesy of Professor D Thurston, University of London.)

Molecular mechanics also enables the medicinal chemist to calculate the binding energy of a ligand. This is the energy **lost** when the ligand binds to its target site, that is

$$E_{binding} = E_{target} + E_{ligand} - E_{target \; plus \; bound \; ligand} \qquad (5.9)$$

All the quantities on the right hand side of the equation may be calculated using molecular mechanics force fields. However, it should be remembered that in many cases the binding of a drug to its target should be weak, because in most cases it has to be able to leave the target after it has activated that site.

A major problem with docking procedures is that the conformation adopted by a ligand when it binds to its target site will depend on the energy of the molecular environment at that site. This means that, although a ligand may have the right pharmacophore, its global minimum energy conformer is not necessarily the conformation that binds to the target site, that is:

$$\text{global minimum energy conformer} \rightleftharpoons \text{bioactive conformer}$$

However, it is normally assumed that the conformers that bind to target sites will be those with a minimum potential energy. Since molecules may have large numbers of such metastable conformers a number of techniques, such as the Metropolis Monte Carlo method and comparative molecular field analysis (CoMFA), have been developed to determine the effect of conformational changes on the effectiveness of docking procedures.

Docking proceedures have also been adapted to design possible leads. The computer is used to fit suitable structural fragments into the docking area. These fragments are joined to make molecules that fit the docking site. This procedure is referred to as **De novo design**.

5.6   Questions

(1)   Describe, by means of notes and sketches, in outline only, the following types of molecular model representation: (i) CPK model, (ii) ball and stick model and (iii) ribbon structure.

(2)   (a) Describe the assumptions that form the basis of the molecular mechanics approach to molecular modelling.

      (b) What is meant by the term force field?

      (c) Construct an expression for $E_{Coulombic}$ for a molecule of ethane ignoring all the possible long range interactions.

(continued)

    (d) What are the advantages and disadvantages of using molecular mechanics to model molecular structures?

(3) Outline the steps you would take in order to create a molecular mechanics model of aspirin.

(4) Explain the significance of the terms: global and local minimum energy conformations.

(5) Describe, in outline only, what is meant by; (a) molecular dynamics and (b) docking.

(6) (a) What is the principle that forms the basis of the quantum mechanical approach to molecular modelling?

    (b) State and name the equation that is the starting point of the wave mechanical approach to molecular modelling.

    (c) What are the major advantages and disadvantages of the quantum mechanical approach to molecular modelling?

6 Combinatorial chemistry

6.1 Introduction

The rapid increase in molecular biology technology has resulted in the development of rapid efficient drug testing systems. The techniques used by these systems are collectively known as **high throughput screening**. High throughput screening methods give accurate results even when extremely small amounts of the test substance are available. However, if it is to be used in an economic fashion as well as efficiently this technology requires the rapid production of a large number of substances for testing, which cannot be met by the stepwise approach of traditional organic synthesis methods (Figure 6.1).

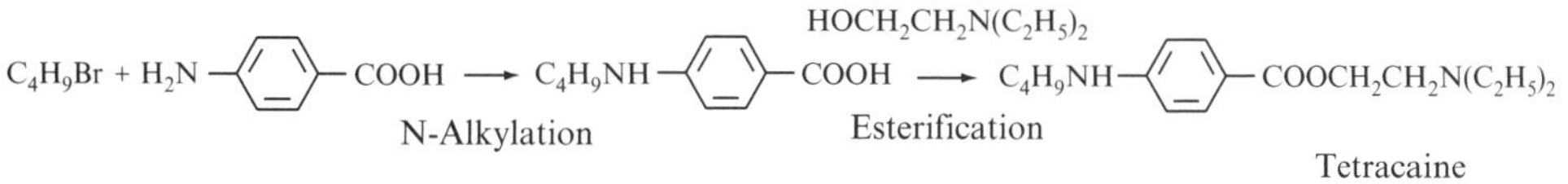

$$C_4H_9Br + H_2N \text{—} \langle \bigcirc \rangle \text{— COOH} \xrightarrow[\text{N-Alkylation}]{} C_4H_9NH \text{—} \langle \bigcirc \rangle \text{— COOH} \xrightarrow[\text{Esterification}]{HOCH_2CH_2N(C_2H_5)_2} C_4H_9NH \text{—} \langle \bigcirc \rangle \text{— COOCH_2CH_2N(C_2H_5)_2}$$

Tetracaine

Figure 6.1 A traditional stepwise organic synthesis scheme illustrated by the synthesis of the local anaesthetic tetracaine

Combinatorial chemistry was developed to produce the large numbers of compounds required for high throughput screening. It allows the simultaneous synthesis of a large number of the possible compounds that could be formed from a number of building blocks. The products of such a process are known as a **combinatorial library**. Libraries may be a collection of individual compounds or mixtures of compounds. Screening the components of a library for activity using high throughput screening techniques enables the development team to select suitable compounds for a more detailed investigation by either combinatorial chemistry or other methods.

The basic concept of combinatorial chemistry is best illustrated by an example. Consider, the reaction of a set of three compounds (A_{1-3}) with a set of three building blocks (B_{1-3}). In combinatorial synthesis, A_1 would simultaneously

Fundamentals of Medicinal Chemistry, Edited by Gareth Thomas
© 2003 John Wiley & Sons, Ltd
ISBN 0 470 84306 3 (Hbk), ISBN 0 470 84307 1 (pbk)

undergo separate reactions with compounds B_1, B_2 and B_3 respectively (Figure 6.2). At the same time compounds A_2 and A_3 would also be undergoing

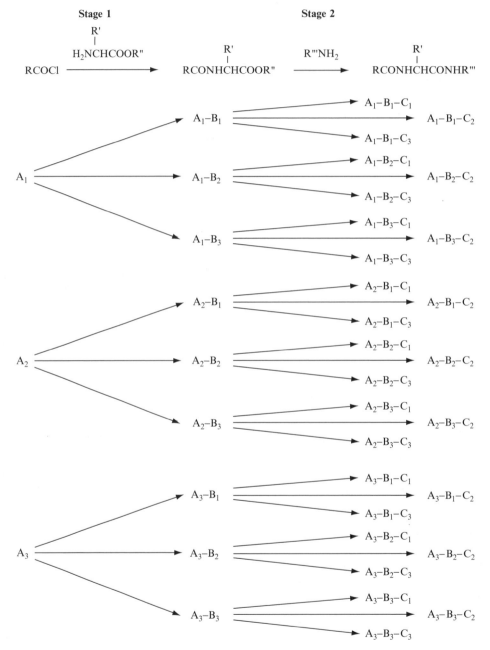

Figure 6.2 The principle of combinatorial chemistry illustrated by a scheme for synthesis of a library of 27 polyamides using three building blocks at each stage

reactions with compounds B_1, B_2 and B_3. These simultaneous reactions would produce a library of nine products. If this process is repeated by reacting these nine products with three new building blocks (C_{1-3}) a combinatorial library of 27 new products would be obtained.

The reactions used at each stage in such a synthesis normally involve the same functional groups, that is, the same type of reaction occurs in each case. Very few libraries have been constructed where different types of reaction are involved in the same stage. In theory this approach results in the formation of all the possible products that could be formed. However, in practice some reactions may not occur.

6.1.1   The design of combinatorial syntheses

One of two general strategies may be followed when designing a combinatorial synthesis (Figure 6.3(a)). In the first case the building blocks are successively added to the preceding structure so that it grows in only one direction. It usually relies on the medicinal chemist finding suitable protecting groups so that the reactions are selective. This design approach is useful if the product is a polymer (**oligomer**) formed from a small number of monomeric units. Alternatively, the synthesis can proceed in different directions from an initial building block known as a **template**, provided the template has either the necessary functional groups or they can be generated during the course of the synthesis (Figure 6.3(b)). Both routes may require the use of protecting groups.

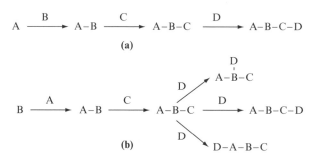

Figure 6.3   (a) The sequential attachment of building blocks. (b) The non-sequential attachment of building blocks using B as a template

The reactions used when designing a combinatorial sequence should *ideally* satisfy the following criteria:

1. the reactions should be specific, relatively easy to carry out and give a high yield;

2. the reactions used in the sequence should allow for the formation of as wide a range of structures for the final products as possible, including all the possible stereoisomers;

3. the reactions should be suitable for use in automated equipment;

4. the building blocks should be readily available;

5. the building blocks should be as diverse as possible so that the range of final products includes structures that utilize all the types of bonding to bind to or react with the target and

6. it must be possible to accurately determine the structures of the final products.

In practice, it is not always possible to select reactions that meet all these criteria. However, condition 6 must be satisfied, otherwise there is little point in carrying out the synthesis.

The degree of information available about the intended target will also influence the selection of the building blocks. If little is known, a random selection of building blocks is used in order to identify a lead. However, if a there is a known lead, the building blocks are selected so that they produce analogues that are related to the structure of the lead. This allows the investigator to study the SAR and/or determine the optimum structure for potency.

6.1.2 The general techniques used in combinatorial synthesis

Combinatorial synthesis may be carried out on a solid support (see section 6.2) or in solution (see section 6.4). In both cases synthesis usually proceeds using one of the strategies outlined in Figure 6.3. Both solid support and solution synthetic methods may be used to produce libraries that consist of either individual compounds or mixtures of compounds. Each type of synthetic method has its own distinct advantages and disadvantages (Table 6.1).

Table 6.1   A comparison of the advantages and disadvantages of the solid support and in solution techniques of combinatorial chemistry

On a solid support	In solution
Reagents can be used in excess in order to drive the reaction to completion	Reagents cannot be used in excess, unless addition purification is carried out
Purification is easy: simply wash the support	Purification can be difficult
Automation is easy	Automation is difficult
Fewer suitable reactions	In theory any organic reaction can be used
Scale-up relatively expensive	Scale-up is easy and relatively inexpensive
Not well documented and time will be required to find a suitable support and linker for a specific synthesis	Only requires time for the development of the chemistry

6.2   The solid support method

The solid support method originated with Merrifields solid support peptide synthesis. It uses resin beads that have a large number of functional groups attached to the surface by a variety of structures known as either a **handle** or a **linker** (Figure 6.4). Each of these functional groups acts as the starting point for the synthesis of one molecule of a product. Since a bead will possess in the order of 6×10^3 functional groups of the same type the amount of the product formed on one bead is often sufficient for structure determination and high throughput screening.

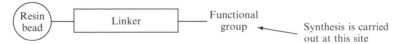

Figure 6.4   A schematic representation of the resin beads used in combinatorial synthesis

The linker moves the point of substrate attachment away from the surface of the bead. This has the effect of reducing steric hindrance, thereby making reaction easier. The choice of linker will depend on the nature of the reactions used in the proposed synthetic pathway (Figure 6.5). For example, an acid labile linker, such as HMP (hydroxymethylphenoxy resin), would not be suitable if the reaction pathway contained reactions that were conducted under strongly acidic conditions. Consideration must also be given to the ease of detaching the product from the linker at the end of the synthesis. The method employed must not damage the required product but must also lend itself to automation.

In 1985 Houghton introduced his **tea bag** method for the rapid solid phase multiple peptide synthesis. In this technique the beads are contained within a porous polypropylene bag. All the reactions, including deprotections, are

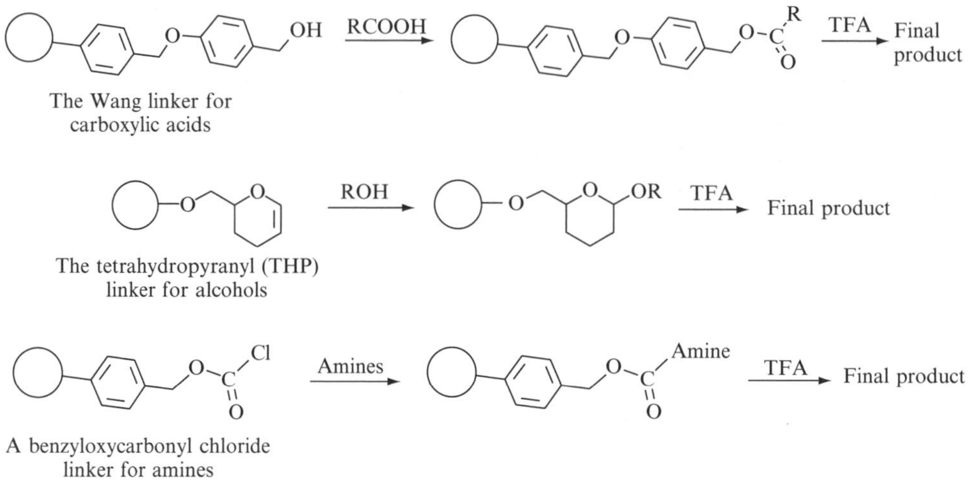
OH
RCOOH
O-C
R
O
TFA
Final product
The Wang linker for carboxylic acids
ROH
OR
TFA
Final product
The tetrahydropyranyl (THP) linker for alcohols
Cl
Amines
Amine
TFA
Final product
A benzyloxycarbonyl chloride linker for amines

Figure 6.5 Examples of linkers that use trifluoroacetic acid (TFA) to detach the final product

carried out by placing the bags in solutions containing the appropriate reagents. The use of the bag makes it easy to purify the resin beads by washing with the appropriate solutions. Furthermore, the method has considerable flexibility and has been partly automated.

Combinatorial synthesis on solid supports is usually carried out by using either the parallel synthesis (see section 6.2.1) or the Furka split and mix procedures (see section 6.2.2). The precise method and approach adopted when using these methods will depend on the nature of the combinatorial library being produced and also the objectives of the investigating team. However, in all cases it is necessary to determine the structures of the components of the library by either keeping a detailed record of the steps involved in the synthesis or giving beads a label that can be decoded to give the structure of the compound attached to that bead (see section 6.3). The method adopted to identify the components of the library will depend on the nature of the synthesis.

6.2.1 Parallel synthesis

In parallel synthesis the compounds are prepared in separate reaction vessels but at the same time, that is, in parallel. The array of individual reaction vessels often takes the form of either a grid of wells in a plastic plate or a grid of plastic rods called pins attached to a plastic base plate (Figure 6.6) that fits into a corresponding set of wells. In the former case the synthesis is carried out on beads placed in the wells whilst in the latter case it takes place on so called

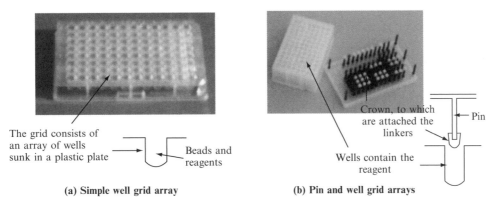

The grid consists of an array of wells sunk in a plastic plate — Beads and reagents

Crown, to which are attached the linkers — Pin

Wells contain the reagent

(a) Simple well grid array   **(b) Pin and well grid arrays**

Figure 6.6 Examples of the arrays used in combinatorial chemical synthesis

plastic 'crowns' pushed on to the tops of the pins, the building blocks being attached to these crowns by linkers similar to those found on the resin beads. The position of each synthetic pathway in the array and hence the structure of the product of that pathway is usually identified by a grid code.

The technique of parallel synthesis is best illustrated by means of an example. Consider the general theoretical steps that would be necessary for the preparation of a combinatorial library of hydantoins by the reaction of isocyanates with amino acids (Figure 6.7) using a 96 well array.

Eight N-protected amino acids (X1, X2, ... X8) are placed in the well array so that only one type of amino acid occupies a row, that is row A will only contain amino acid X1, row B will only contain amino acid X2 and so on (Figure 6.8(a)). Beads are added to each well and the array placed in a reaction environment that will join the X compound to the linker of the bead. The amino acids are deprotected by hydrogenolysis and 12 isocyanates (Y1, Y2, ..., Y8) added to the wells so that each numbered row at right angles to the lettered rows contains only one type of isocyanate. In other words, compound Y1 is only added to row one, compound Y2 is only added to row two and so on (Figure 6.8(b)). The isocyanates are allowed to react to form substituted ureas, which

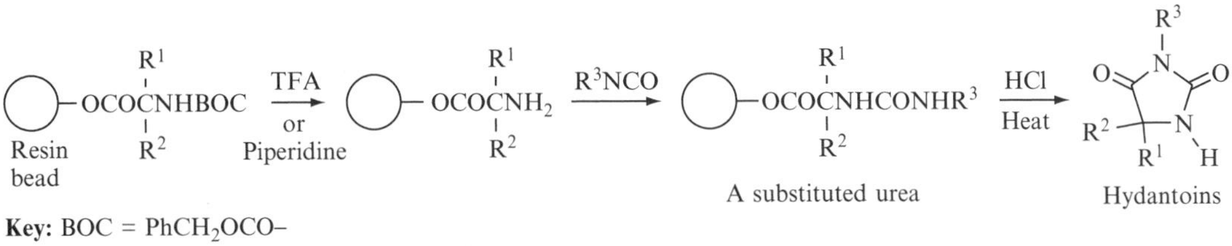

Resin bead $-OCOC\overset{R^1}{\underset{R^2}{|}}NHBOC$ $\xrightarrow[\text{Piperidine}]{\text{TFA or}}$ $-OCOC\overset{R^1}{\underset{R^2}{|}}NH_2$ $\xrightarrow{R^3NCO}$ $-OCOC\overset{R^1}{\underset{R^2}{|}}NHCONHR^3$ $\xrightarrow[\text{Heat}]{\text{HCl}}$ Hydantoins

A substituted urea

Key: BOC = PhCH$_2$OCO–

Figure 6.7 The reaction of amino acids with isocyanates to form hydantoins

	A	B	C	D	E	F	G	H
1	X1	X2	X3	X4	X5	X6	X7	X8
2	X1	X2	X3	X4	X5	X6	X7	X8
3	X1	X2	X3	X4	X5	X6	X7	X8
4	X1	X2	X3	X4	X5	X6	X7	X8
5	X1	X2	X3	X4	X5	X6	X7	X8
6	X1	X2	X3	X4	X5	X6	X7	X8
7	X1	X2	X3	X4	X5	X6	X7	X8
8	X1	X2	X3	X4	X5	X6	X7	X8
9	X1	X2	X3	X4	X5	X6	X7	X8
10	X1	X2	X3	X4	X5	X6	X7	X8
11	X1	X2	X3	X4	X5	X6	X7	X8
12	X1	X2	X3	X4	X5	X6	X7	X8

Deprotection of the amino acid →

	A	B	C	D	E	F	G	H
1	X1–Y1	X2–Y1	X3–Y1	X4–Y1	X5–Y1	X6–Y1	X7–Y1	X8–Y1
2	X1–Y2	X2–Y2	X3–Y2	X4–Y2	X5–Y2	X6–Y2	X7–Y2	X8–Y2
3	X1–Y3	X2–Y3	X3–Y3	X4–Y3	X5–Y3	X6–Y3	X7–Y3	X8–Y3
4	X1–Y4	X2–Y4	X3–Y4	X4–Y4	X5–Y4	X6–Y4	X7–Y4	X8–Y4
5	X1–Y5	X2–Y5	X3–Y5	X4–Y5	X5–Y5	X6–Y5	X7–Y5	X8–Y5
6	X1–Y6	X2–Y6	X3–Y6	X4–Y6	X5–Y6	X6–Y6	X7–Y6	X8–Y6
7	X1–Y7	X2–Y7	X3–Y7	X4–Y7	X5–Y7	X6–Y7	X7–Y7	X8–Y7
8	X1–Y8	X2–Y8	X3–Y8	X4–Y8	X5–Y8	X6–Y8	X7–Y8	X8–Y8
9	X1–Y9	X2–Y9	X3–Y9	X4–Y9	X5–Y9	X6–Y9	X7–Y9	X8–Y9
10	X1–Y10	X2–Y10	X3–Y10	X4–Y10	X5–Y10	X6–Y10	X7–Y10	X8–Y10
11	X1–Y11	X2–Y11	X3–Y11	X4–Y11	X5–Y11	X6–Y11	X7–Y11	X8–Y11
12	X1–Y12	X2–Y12	X3–Y12	X4–Y12	X5–Y12	X6–Y12	X7–Y12	X8–Y12

(a) The placement of the first building blocks, the BOC protected amino acids X1 to X12 and their attachment to the resin

(b) The placement of the isocyanate building blocks Y1 to Y8

The hydantoins Z1 to Z96

	A	B	C	D	E	F	G	H
1	Z1	Z2	Z3	Z4	Z5	Z6	Z7	Z8
2	Z9	Z10	Z11	Z12	Z13	Z14	Z15	Z16
3	Z17	Z18	Z19	Z20	Z21	Z22	Z23	Z24
4	Z25	Z26	Z27	Z28	Z29	Z30	Z31	Z32
5	Z33	Z34	Z35	Z36	Z37	Z38	Z39	Z40
6	Z41	Z42	Z43	Z44	Z45	Z46	Z47	Z48
7	Z49	Z50	Z51	Z52	Z53	Z54	Z55	Z56
8	Z57	Z58	Z59	Z60	Z61	Z62	Z63	Z64
9	Z65	Z66	Z67	Z68	Z69	Z70	Z71	Z72
10	Z73	Z74	Z75	Z76	Z77	Z78	Z79	Z80
11	Z81	Z82	Z83	Z84	Z85	Z86	Z87	Z88
12	Z89	Z90	Z91	Z92	Z93	Z94	Z95	Z96

(c) Reaction, by placing the array in a suitable eaction environment, to form the substituted urea and subsequent treatment with hot 6M hydrochloric acid to form the hydantoins Z1 to Z96

Figure 6.8 The pattern of well loading for the formation of a combinatorial library of 96 hydantoins

are attached to the beads via the linker. The array is washed with suitable reagents to purify the ureas. Each well is treated with 6 M hydrochloric acid and the whole array heated to simultaneously form the hydantoins and release them from the resin. Although it is possible to simultaneously synthesize a total of 96 different hydantoins (Z1–Z96, Figure 6.8(c)) by this technique, in practice it is likely that some of the reactions will be unsuccessful and a somewhat smaller library of compounds would normally be obtained.

A well array combinatorial synthesis can consist of any number of stages. Each stage is carried out in the general manner described for the previous example. However, at each stage only either the numbered or lettered rows are used, not both, unless a library of mixtures is required. Finally, the products are liberated from the resin by the appropriate linker cleavage reaction (see Figure 6.5)

and the products isolated. The structures of these products are usually determined by following the history of the synthesis using the grid references of the
wells and confirmed by instrumental methods (mainly NMR, GC, HPLC
and MS).

The pin array is used in a similar manner to the well array except the array of
crowns is inverted so that the crowns are suspended in the reagents placed in a
corresponding array of wells (Figure 6.6(b)). Reaction is brought about
by placing the combined pin and well unit in a suitable reaction environment.
The loading of the wells follows the pattern described in Figure 6.8. The parallel
and pin methods are not the only solid support methods of obtaining combinatorial libraries. A number of other techniques using solid supports have also
been developed.

6.2.2 Furka's mix and split technique

The Furka method produces the library of compounds on resin beads. It may be
used to make both large (thousands) and small (hundreds) combinatorial libraries. Large libraries are possible because the technique produces one type of
compound on each bead, that is, all the molecules formed on one bead are the
same but different from those formed on all the other beads. Each bead will
yield up to 6×10^{13} product molecules, which is sufficient to carry out high
throughput screening procedures. The technique has the advantage that it
reduces the number of reactions required to produce a large library.

The beads are divided into a number of equally sized portions corresponding
to the number of initial building blocks. Each starting compound is attached to
its own group of beads using the appropriate chemical reaction (Figure 6.9). All
the portions of beads are now mixed and separated into the number of equal
portions corresponding to the number of different starting compounds being
used for the first stage of the synthesis. One reactant building block is added to
each portion and the reaction carried out by putting the mixtures of resin beads
and reactants in a suitable reaction vessel. After reaction all the beads are mixed
before separating them into the number of equal portions corresponding to
the number of reactants being used in the second stage of the synthesis. One
of the second stage building blocks is added to each of these new portions and the
mixture allowed to react to produce the products for this stage in the synthesis.
This process of mix and split is continued until the required library is synthesized. In peptide and similar polymer library formation where the same building
blocks are used at each step, the maximum possible number of compounds

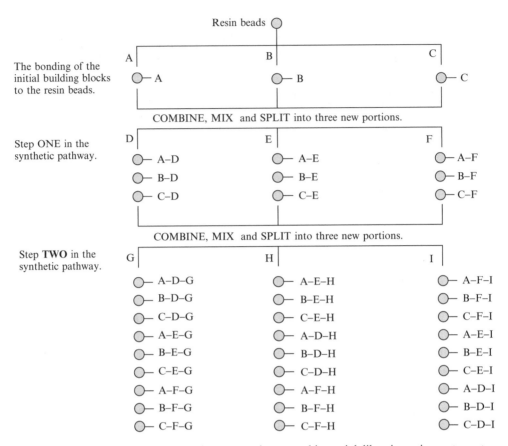

Figure 6.9 An example of the Furka approach to combinatorial libraries using a two step synthesis involving three building blocks at each stage

that can be synthesized for a given number of different building blocks (b) is given by:

$$\text{number of compounds} = b^x \qquad (6.1)$$

where x is the number of steps in the synthesis.

Unlike in parallel synthesis the history of the bead cannot be traced from a grid reference; it has to be traced using a suitable encoding method (see section 6.3) or deconvolution (see section 6.5). Encoding methods use a code to indicate what has happened at each step in the synthesis. They range from putting an identifiable tag compound on to the bead at each step in the synthesis to using computer readable silicon chips as the solid support. If sufficient compound is produced its identity may also be confirmed using a combination of analytical methods such as NMR, MS, HPLC and GC.

6.3   Encoding methods

A wide variety of encoding methods have been developed to record the history of a bead used in the Furka mix and split technique. This section outlines some of these methods.

6.3.1   Sequential chemical tagging methods

Sequential chemical tagging methods uses specific compounds (tags) as a code for the individual steps in the synthesis. These tag compounds are sequentially attached in the form of a polymer-like molecule to the same linker or bead as the library compound at each step in the synthesis (Figure 6.10). The amount of tag used at each step must be strictly controlled so that only a very small percentage of the available linker functional groups are occupied by a tag. At the end of the synthesis both the library compound and the tag compound are liberated from the bead. The tag compound must be produced in a sufficient amount to enable it to be decoded to give the history and hence the possible structure of the library compound.

Compounds used for tagging must satisfy a number of criteria:

1. the concentration of the tag should be just sufficient for its analysis, that is, the majority of the linkers should be occupied by the combinatorial synthesis;

2. the tagging reaction must take place under conditions that are compatible with those used for the synthesis of the library compound;

3. it must be possible to separate the tag from the library compound and

4. analysis of the tag should be rapid and accurate, using methods that could be automated.

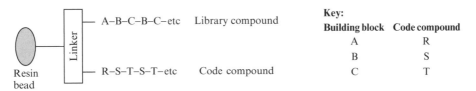

Figure 6.10   Chemical encoding of resin beads. Branched linkers, with one site for attaching the library compound and another for attaching the tag, are often used for encoding

Table 6.2 The use of oligonucleotides to encode amino acids in peptide synthesis

Amino acid	Structure	Oligonucleotide code
Glycine (Gly)	$\underset{\displaystyle CH_2COOH}{\overset{\displaystyle NH_2}{\vert}}$	CACATG
Methionine (Met)	$CH_3SCH_2CH_2\underset{\displaystyle}{\overset{\displaystyle NH_2}{\underset{\vert}{C}}}HCOOH$	ACGGTA

Many peptide libraries have been encoded using single stranded DNA oligo-nucleotides as tags. Each oligonucleotide acts as the code for one amino acid (Table 6.2). Furthermore, a polymerase chain reaction (PCR) primer is usually attached to the tag site so that at the end of the combinatorial synthesis the concentration of the completed tag DNA-oligonucleotide molecule may be increased using the *Taq* polymerase procedure. This amplification of the yield of the tag makes it easier to identify the sequence of bases, which leads to a more accurate decoding.

At each stage in the peptide synthesis a second parallel synthesis is carried out on the same bead to attach the oligonucleotide tag (Figure 6.11). In other words, two alternating parallel syntheses are carried out at the same time. On comple-tion of the peptide synthesis, the oligonucleotide tag is isolated from the bead and its base sequence determined and decoded to give the sequence of amino acid residues in the peptide.

Peptides have also been used as tags (Figure 6.12) in a similar manner to DNA oligo nucleotides. The sequence of amino acids in the encoding peptide is determined using the Edman sequencing method. This amino acid sequence is used to determine the history of the formation and hence the structure of the product found on that bead.

6.3.2 Still's binary code tag system

A unique approach by Still was to give each building block its own chemical equivalent of a binary code for each stage of the synthesis using inert aryl halides (Figure 6.13(a)). One or more of these tags are directly attached to the resin using a photolabile linker at the appropriate points in the synthesis. They indicate the nature of the building block and the stage at which it was incorpor-ated into the solid support (Table 6.3). Aryl halide tags are used because they can be detected in very small amounts by GC. They are selected on the basis that their retention times are roughly equally spaced (Figure 6.13(b)). At the end of

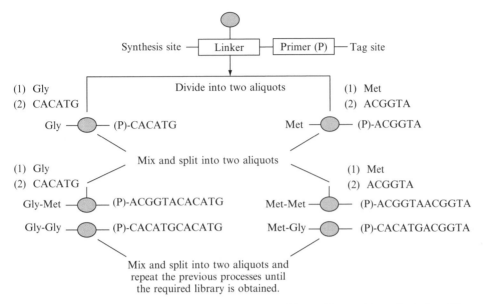

Figure 6.11 The use of oligonucleotides to encode a peptide combinatorial synthesis for a library based on two building blocks

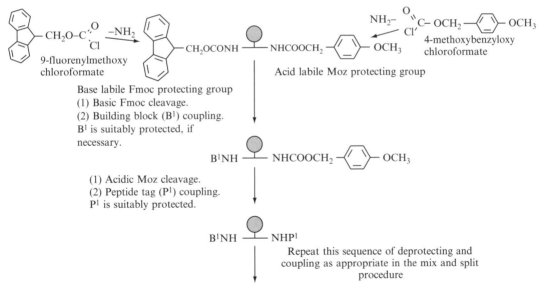

Figure 6.12 An outline of the Zuckermann approach using peptides for encoding

the synthesis all the tags are detached from the linker and are detected by GC. The gas chromatogram is read like a bar code to account for the history of the bead. Suppose, for example, that the formation of a tripeptide using six aryl

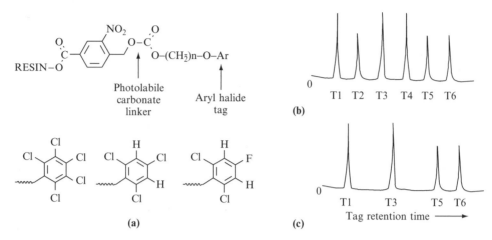

Figure 6.13 (a) Molecular tags used by Still. ᴡᴡᴡᴡ-Indicates the point at which the tag is attached to the linker. (b) A hypothetical representation of the GC plots obtained for some aryl halide tags T_1 to T_6. (c) The tag chromatogram for a hypothetical tagging scheme.

Table 6.3 A hypothetical tagging scheme for the preparation of tripeptides using binary combinations of six tags

	Tag		
Stage	Glycine (Gly)	Alanine (Ala)	Serine (Ser)
1	T1	T2	T1+T2
2	T3	T4	T3+T4
3	T5	T6	T5+T6

halide tags allocated as shown in the tagging scheme outlined in Table 6.3 gave the tag chromatogram shown in Figure 6.13(b). The presence of T1 shows that in the first stage of the synthesis the first amino acid residue is glycine. This residue will be attached via its the C-terminus of the peptide if a linker with an amino group was used and its N-terminus if a linker with an acid group was used. The presence of T3 shows that the second residue is also glycine, whilst the presence of T5 and T6 indicates that the third amino acid in the peptide is serine.

6.3.3 Computerized tagging

Nicolaou has devised a method of using silicon chips to record the history of a synthesis. Silicon chips can be coded to receive and store radio signals in the form of a binary code. This code can be used as a code for the building blocks of a synthesis. The silicon chip and beads are placed in a container known as a **can** that is porous to the reagents used in the synthesis. Each can is closed and treated as though it were one bead in a mix and split synthesis. The cans are divided into the required number of aliquots corresponding to the number of building blocks used in the initial step of the synthesis. Each batch of cans is reacted with its own building block and the chip is irradiated with the appropriate radio signal for that building block. The mix and split procedure is followed and at each step the chips in the batch are irradiated with the appropriate radio signal. At the end of the synthesis the prepared library compound is cleaved from the chip, which is interrogated to determine the history of the compound synthesized on the chip. The method has the advantage of producing larger amounts of the required compounds than the normal mix and split approach because the same compound is produced on all the beads in a can.

6.4 Combinatorial synthesis in solution

The main problem with preparing libraries using solution chemistry is the difficulty of removing unwanted impurities at each step in the synthesis. Consequently, many of the strategies used for the preparation of libraries using solution chemistry are directed to the purification of the products of each steps of the synthesis. This and other practical problems has usually restricted the use of solution combinatorial chemistry to synthetic pathways consisting of two or three steps.

Combinatorial synthesis in solution can be used to produce libraries that consist of single compounds or mixtures using traditional organic chemistry. Single compound libraries are prepared using the parallel synthesis technique (see section 6.2.1). Libraries of mixtures are formed by separately reacting each of the members of a set of similar compounds with the same mixture of all the members of the second set of compounds. Consider, for example, a combinatorial library of amides formed by reacting a set of five acid chlorides (A^1–A^5) with ten amines (B^1–B^{10}). Each of the five acid chlorides is reacted separately with an equimolar mixture of all ten amines and each of the amines is reacted with an equimolar mixture of all the acid chlorides (Figure 6.14). This produces a library consisting of a set of five mixtures based on individual acid halides and 10 mixtures based on individual amines. This means that each compound in the library is prepared twice, once from the acid chloride set and once from the amine set. Consequently, determining the most biologically active of the mixtures from the acid halide set will define the acyl part of the most active amide and similarly identifying the most biologically active of the amine based

$$RCOCl + R'NH2 \longrightarrow RCONHR' + Cl$$

The acid chloride based set:

$A^1 + (B^1,B^2,B^3,B^4,B^5,B^6,B^7,B^8,B^9,B^{10}) \longrightarrow$ **Mixture 1** containing all the possible A^1–B compounds.

$A^2 + (B^1,B^2,B^3,B^4,B^5,B^6,B^7,B^8,B^9,B^{10}) \longrightarrow$ **Mixture 2** containing all the possible A^2–B compounds.

$\vdots$ Etc. $\vdots$ Etc.

$A^5 + (B^1,B^2,B^3,B^4,B^5,B^6,B^7,B^8,B^9,B^{10}) \longrightarrow$ **Mixture 5** containing all the possible A^5–B compounds.

The amine based set:

$B^1 + (A^1,A^2,A^3,A^4,A^5,) \longrightarrow$ **Mixture 6** containing all the possible B^1–A compounds.

$\vdots$ Etc. $\vdots$ Etc.

$B^{10} + (A^1,A^2,A^3,A^4,A^5,) \longrightarrow$ **Mixture 15** containing all the possible B^1–A compounds.

Figure 6.14 A schematic representation of the index approach to identifying active compounds in libraries formed in solution

set of mixtures will identify the amine residue of that amide. Libraries used in this manner are often referred to as indexed libraries.

This method of identifying the structure of the most active component of combinatorial libraries of mixtures is known as **deconvolution** (see section 6.5). It depends on both the mixtures containing the active compound giving a positive result for the assay procedure. It is not possible to identify the active structure if one of the sets of mixtures gives a negative result. Furthermore, complications arise if more than one mixture is found to be active. In this case all the possible structures have to be synthesized and tested separately. However, it is generally found that the activities of the library mixtures are usually higher than those exhibited by the individual compounds responsible for activity after they have been isolated from the mixture.

6.5   Screening and deconvolution

The success of a library depends not only on it containing the right compounds but also on the efficiency of the screening procedure. Furthermore, it is no use preparing a combinatorial library if there is not a suitable screening procedure

to assess the components of the library. A key problem with very large combinatorial libraries of mixtures is the large amount of work required to screen
these libraries.

Deconvolution is a method, based on the process of elimination, of reducing
the number of screening tests required to locate the most active member of a
library consisting of a mixture of all the components. It is based on producing
and biologically assaying similar secondary libraries that contain one less building block than the original library. It is emphasized that the biological assay is
carried out on a mixture of all the members of the secondary library. If the
secondary library is still as active as the original library the missing building
block is not part of the active structure. Repetition of this process will eventually
result in a library that is inactive, which indicates that the missing building block
in this library is part of the active structure. This procedure is carried out for
each of the building blocks at each step in the synthesis. Suppose, for example,
one has a tripeptide library consisting of a mixture of 1000 compounds. This
library was produced from 10 different amino acids (A^1–A^{10}) using two synthetic steps, each of which involved 10 building blocks (Figure 6.15). The
formation of a secondary library by omitting amino acid A^1 from the initial
set of amino acids but reacting these nine with all 10 amino acids in the first and
second steps would produce 900 compounds. These compounds will not contain
amino acid residue A^1 in the first position of the tripeptide. If the resulting
library is biologically inactive the active compound must contain the residue at
position one in the tripeptide. However, if the mixture is active the process must
be repeated using A^1 but omitting a different amino acid residue from the
synthesis. In the worst scenario it would mean that the 900 member library
would have to be prepared ten times in order to determine first residue of
the most active tripeptide. Repeating this process of omission, combinatorial

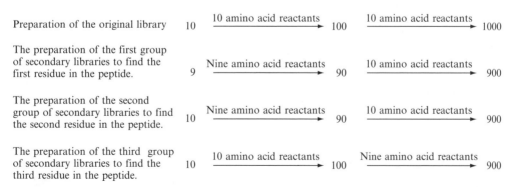

Figure 6.15 A schematic representation of convolution. The figures indicate the number of
components in the mixture

synthesis and biological testing but using groups of nine reactants for the first step will give the amino acid that occupies the second place in the peptide chain. Further repetition but using groups of nine amino acid reactants in the second step will identify the third amino acid in the chain.

In order to be effective, deconvolution procedures require that both the synthesis and assay of the library be rapid. The procedure is complicated when there is more than one active component in the library. In this case it is necessary to prepare and test all the possible compounds indicated by deconvolution in order to identify the most active compound in the library.

6.6   Questions

(1)   Outline the basic principle underlying combinatorial chemistry. What criteria should be satisfied by the building blocks used in a combinatorial synthesis?

(2)   List the general considerations that should be taken into account when designing a combinatorial synthesis.

(3)   Outline the parallel synthesis technique for carrying out a combinatorial synthesis. How does this method differ from Furka's mix and split method?

(4)
$$\overset{R^1}{\underset{|}{}}\quad\overset{R^2}{\underset{|}{}}$$
H$_2$NCHCONHCHCOOH

   (B)

   Outline a design for a combinatorial synthesis for the formation of a combinatorial library of nine compounds with the general formula B using the Furka mix and split method. Outline any essential practical details. Details of the chemistry of peptide link formation are not required; it is sufficient to say that it is formed.

(5)   Outline the range of encoding methods used to deduce the structures of compounds produced in a Furka mix and split combinatorial synthesis.

(6)   Describe, in general terms, how the technique of deconvolution can be used to identify the most active component in a combinatorial library consisting of groups of mixtures of compounds.

7 Selected Examples of Drug Action at Some Common Target Areas

7.1 Introduction

The action of drugs and the sites at which they are believed to act are very varied. Common target sites are the cell envelopes and walls of microorganisms, enzymes, receptors, nucleic acids and viruses. This chapter describes the structures and outlines the action of some of the drugs that target these sites. It also outlines some of the general strategies adopted to discover new leads for some of these targets.

7.2 Examples of drugs that disrupt cell membranes and walls

Cells are broadly classified as either **eukaryotes** or **prokaryotes** (see Appendix 3). Both types have a membrane, known as the **cytoplasmic** or **plasma membrane** (see Appendix 3), that separates the internal medium (**intracellular fluid**) of the cell from the external medium (**extracellular fluid**). Cytoplasmic membranes may also divide the interior of a cell into separate compartments. In addition to the cytoplasmic membrane, the more fragile membranes of plants and bacteria are also protected by a rigid external covering known as a cell wall. The combination of cell wall and plasma membrane is referred to as the **cell envelope** (Appendix 2).

The structure of a cytoplasmic membrane is complex (see Appendix 3). Built into the membrane are receptors (see Appendix 4), enzymes (see Appendix 7)

Fundamentals of Medicinal Chemistry, Edited by Gareth Thomas
© 2003 John Wiley & Sons, Ltd
ISBN 0 470 84306 3 (Hbk), ISBN 0 470 84307 1 (pbk)

and numerous channels connecting the intracellular fluid with the extracellular fluid. These channels allow ions and other small molecules to travel from the interior of the cell to its exterior and vice versa. Those whose primary function is the transport of ions are known as **ion channels**.

Most drugs act on the receptors and enzymes found in cell envelopes. However, a number of drugs act by either disrupting the structure of the cell membranes and walls or inhibiting the formation of cell membranes and walls or blocking ion channels. In general, drugs acting on microorganisms by either disrupting the structures of membranes and walls or their synthesis appear to act by

1. inhibiting the action of enzymes and other substances in the cell membrane involved in the production of compounds necessary for maintaining the integrity of the cell membrane,

2. inhibiting processes involved in the formation of the cell wall, resulting in an incomplete cell wall, which leads to loss of vital cellular material and subsequent death of the cell,

3. forming channels through the cell wall or membrane, making it more porous, which also results in the loss of vital cellular material and the death of the cell, and

4. making the cell more porous by breaking down sections of the membrane.

All microorganisms have plasma membranes, which have characteristics in common. Consequently, drugs can act by the same mechanism on quite different classes of microorganism. For example, griseofulvin is both an antifungal and an antibacterial agent (see section 7.2.1 and 7.2.2). Furthermore, the membranes of prokaryotic cells exhibit a number of significantly different characteristics to those of eukaroytic cells. It is these differences that must be exploited by medicinal chemists if they are to find new drugs to treat microbiological infestations.

7.2.1 Antifungal agents

Fungal infections usually involve the skin and mucous membranes of the body. The fungal microorganisms are believed to damage the cell membrane, leading to a loss of essential cellular components. Antifungal agents counter this attack

Table 7.1 Some of the classes of compound that are used as antifungal agents. Note the common structural features.

Class	General structure	Examples
Azoles based on 1,3-diazoles		Clotrimazole Econazole Sulconazole
Azoles based on 1,2,4-triazoles		Terconazole Fluconazole
Allylamines		Naftifine Terbinafine Tolnaftate
Phenols		Hexylresorcinol Chloroxylenol Clioquinol Ciclopirox

by both **fungistatic** and **fungicidal** action. Fungistatic action occurs when the drug prevents the fungus reproducing with the result that it dies out naturally, whilst fungicidal action kills the fungus. The suffixes-*static* and -*cide* or -*cidal* are widely used in other contexes to indicate these general types of action. Some of the fungicides that act by disrupting the integrity of the cell membranes of fungi are listed in Table 7.1.

7.2.1.1 Azoles

Active azoles are usually derivatives of either 1,3-imidazoles or 1,2,4-imadazoles that exhibit fungistatic activity at nanomolar concentration and fungicidal activity at higher micromolar concentrations. Azoles are active against most fungi that infect the skin and mucous membrane as well as some systemic fungal infections, bacteria, protazoa and helminthi species. They are believed to mainly act by inhibiting cytochrome P-450 enzymes, in particular those that are essential for the biosynthesis of ergosterol, the main steroid found in fungual cell membranes. This is thought to result in an accumulation of 14α-methylated sterols, such as lanosterol, in the membrane. These sterols are believed to increase the membrane's permeability, which allows essential cellular contents to leak from the cell, causing ireversible damage and cell death. Azoles also inhibit P-450 oxidases in mammals but far higher concentrations than those required to treat fungi are usually required.

SAR studies have shown that a weakly basic imidazole or 1,2,4-triazole rings substituted only at the N-1 position are essential for activity. The substituent must be lipophilic in character and usually contains one or more five or six membered ring systems, some of which may be attached by an ether, secondary amine or thioether group to the carbon chain. The more potent compounds have two or three aromatic substituents, which are singly or multiply chlorinated or fluorinated at positions 2, 4 and 6. These nonpolar structures give the compounds a high degree of lipophilicity, and hence membrane solubility.

7.2.1.2 Allylamines

Allylamines are synthetic derivatives of 3-aminopropene (Table 7.1) developed from naftifine, the allylamine group appearing to be essential for activity. They are believed to act by inhibiting squalene epoxidase, the enzyme for the squalene epoxidation stage in the biosynthesis of ergosterol in the fungal membrane. This leads to an increase in squalene concentration in the membrane with subsequent loss of membrane integrity, which allows loss of cell contents to occur. Tolnaftate, although it is not an allylamine, appears to act in a similar fashion. However, allylamines do not appear to significantly inhibit the mammalian cholesterol biosynthesis.

Squalene   2,3-Oxidosqualene   Ergosterol

7.2.1.3 Phenols

There are numerous phenolic antifungal agents (Table 7.1). They are believed to destroy sections of the cell membrane, which results in the loss of the cellular components and the death of the cell. The mechanism by which this destruction occurs is not known.

7.2.2 Antibacterial agents

Antibacterial antibiotics normally act by either making the plasma membrane of bacteria more permeable to essential ions and other small molecules by iono-phoric action or by inhibiting cell wall synthesis (see section 7.2.2). Those compounds that act on the plasma membrane also have the ability to pene-trate the cell wall structure (Appendix 3). In both cases, the net result is a loss in the integrity of the bacterial cell envelope, which leads to irreversible cell damage and death.

7.2.2.1 Ionophoric antibiotic action

Ionophores are substances that can penetrate a membrane and increase its permeability to ions. They transport ions in both directions across a membrane. Consequently, they will only reduce the concentration of a specific ion until its concentration is the same on both sides of a membrane. This reduction in the concentration of essential cell components of a microorganism is often sufficient to lead to the distruction of the organism.

Ionophores are classified as either **channel** or **carrier** ionophores. Channel ionophores form channels across the membrane through which ions can diffuse down a concentration gradient. The nature of the channel depends on the ionophore, for example, gramicidin A channels are formed by two gramicidin molecules, N-terminus to N-terminus, each molecule forming a left-handed helix (Figure 7.1(a)). Carrier ionophores pick up an ion on one side of the membrane, transport it across, and release it into the fluid on the other side of the membrane. They usually transport specific ions. For example, valinomycin transports K^+ but not Na^+ Li^+ ions (Figure 7.1(b)).

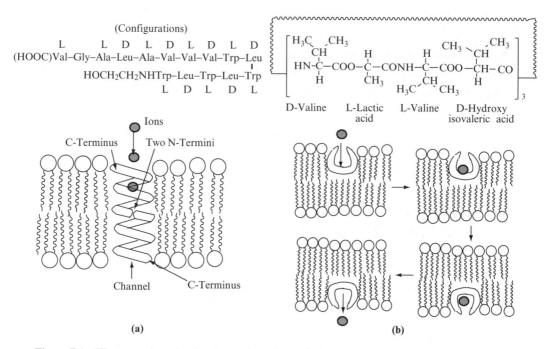

Figure 7.1   The general mode of action of ionophores in ion transport. (a) A channel formed by two gramicidin A molecules, N-terminus to N-terminus. (b) The sequence of events in the operation of a carrier ionophore such as valinomycin. Valinomycin is a cyclic peptide consisting of three repeating units with the structure shown

7.2.2.2   Cell wall synthesis inhibition

The cell walls (Appendix 3) of all bacteria are being continuously replaced because they are continuously being broken down by enzymes in the extracellular fluid. Antibacterial agents, commonly referred to as antibiotics, often act by inhibiting this replacement biosynthesis of the cell wall at any stage in its formation. Most drugs that act in this fashion inhibit either the formation of the precursor starting compounds, the formation of the peptidoglycan chains or the cross linking of the peptidoglycan (Table 7.2). However, increasing numbers of bacteria are resistant to antibiotics, especially to β-lactam antibiotics. This resistance is likely to become a major problem in the future.

The activity of the penicillins and cephalosporins is believed to be due to the β-lactam ring. Bacterial resistance to these drugs is thought to be mainly due to inactivation of the drug by hydrolysis of the β-lactam ring by the β-lactamases produced by the bacteria. Both Gram-positive and Gram-negative bacteria (Appendix 2) produce β-lactamases. In the former case, the enzyme is liberated into the medium surrounding the the bacteria, which results in the hydrolysis of

Table 7.2 Examples of drugs that inhibit the formation of cell wall synthesis

Compound/Active against	Structure	Mode of action
D-Cycloserine. A broad spectrum antibiotic.	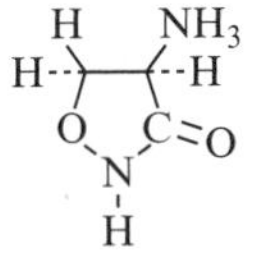 D-Cycloserine 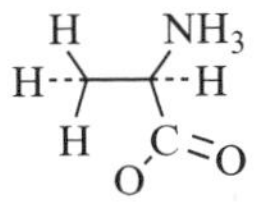 D-Alanine	Inhibits the enzymes alanine racemase and D-alanyl-D-alanyl synthetase that are responsible for producing the dipeptide D-alanyl-D-alanine, a precursor of the pentapeptide chain in cell wall formation. It is believed that the rigid structure of the isoxazole ring gives the drug a better chance of binding to the enzyme than the more flexible structure of D-alanine.
Fosomycin. Active against Gram-positive and Gram-negative bacteria.	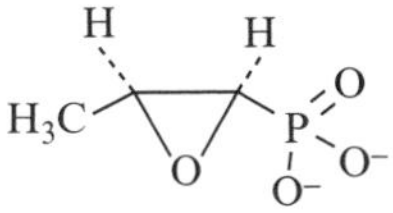 Fosomycin	Inhibits enol-pyruvate transferase, which catalyses the incorporation of phosphoenolpyruvic acid (PEP) into uridine diphospho-N-acetylglucoamine (UDPNAG), a precursor involved in the formation of bacterial cell walls.
Bacitracin A. Active against Gram-positive bacteria. The configurations of the amino acid residues are given in the brackets.	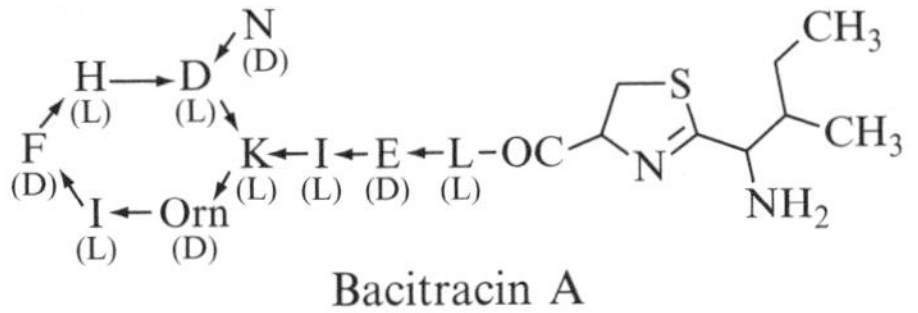 Bacitracin A	Believed to inhibit a number of the stages in the biosynthesis of the peptidoglycan chains. (Letter key, see Table 1.1.)
β-Lactam group of antibiotics. More effective against Gram-positive than Gram-negative bacteria but some cephalosporins, such as ceftazidime, are very effective against Gram-negative bacteria.	Penicillins Cephalosporins	The β-lactam group of antibiotics inhibit cell wall synthesis by inhibiting the formation of the transpeptidases responsible for the cross linking between the peptidoglycan chains.

D-Cycloserine structure labels: H, NH$_3$, H, H, O, C=O, N, H

D-Alanine structure labels: H, NH$_3$, H, H, H, C=O, O

Fosomycin structure labels: H, H, H$_3$C, O, P, O, O⁻, O⁻

Bacitracin A structure labels: N (D), H→D (L), (L), F (D), K←I←E←L-OC (L)(L)(D)(L), I←Orn (L)(D), CH$_3$, S, N, CH$_3$, NH$_2$

Penicillins structure labels: H H, RCONH, S, CH$_3$, CH$_3$, O, N, H COOH

Benzylpenicillin (Penicillin G)

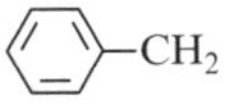

Ampicillin (X = H)
Amoxicillin (X = OH)

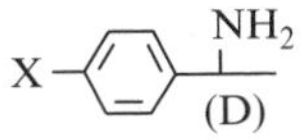

R–

R– for benzylpenicillin: phenyl–CH$_2$

X–phenyl–, NH$_2$, (D)

Cephalothin

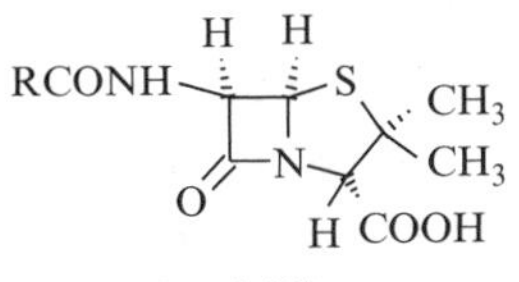

Ceftazidime

Cephalosporins structure labels: H H, RCONH, S, O, N, X, COOH

	R–	X–
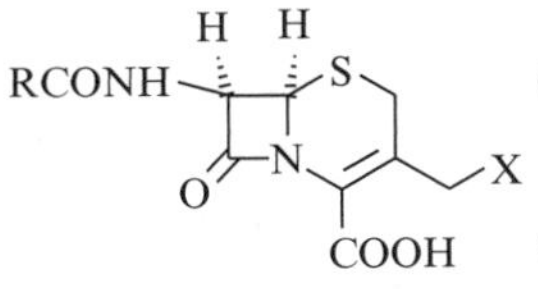 Cephalothin	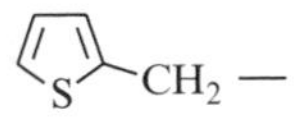 thiophene–CH$_2$–	–OCOCH$_3$
Ceftazidime	HOOCC(CH$_3$)$_2$O, H$_2$N (thiazole) N	–CH$_2$N (pyridine)

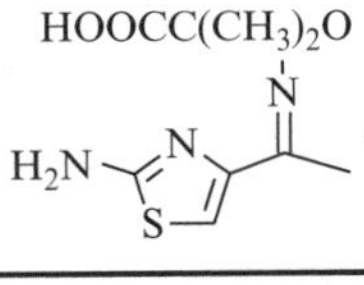

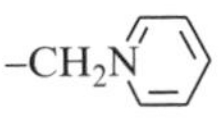

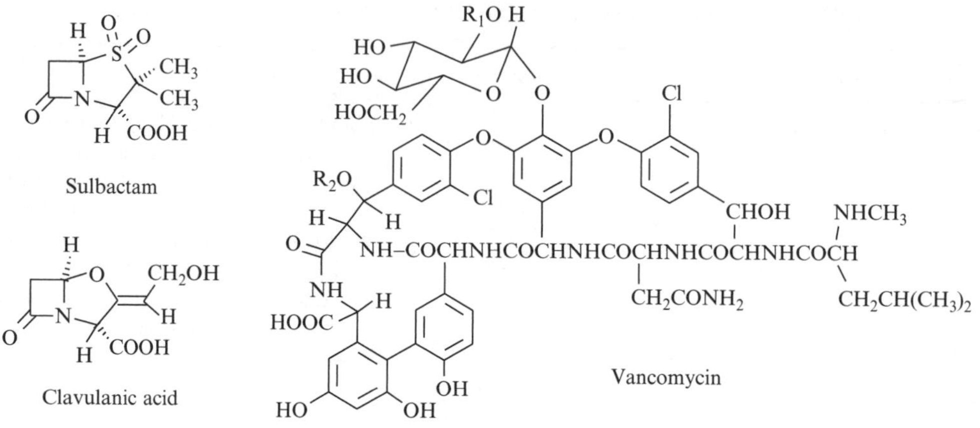

Figure 7.2 (a) β-Lactamase inhibitors and (b) the β-lactamase resistant drug vancomycin

the β-lactam ring before the drug reaches the bacteria. However, with Gram-negative bacteria, the hydrolysis takes place within the periplasmic space. In addition, some Gram-negative bacteria produce *acylases*, which can cleave the side chains of penicillins. Bacteria that have developed a resistance to β-lactam antibiotics are treated using either a dosage form incorporating a β-lactamase inhibitor, such as clavulanic acid or sulbactam, or a lactamase resistant drug, such as vancomycin (Figure 7.2).

7.3 Drugs that target enzymes

Enzymes (Appendix 7) are often targets in drug design. Inhibition offers a method of either preventing or regulating the chemical reactions occuring in pathological conditions. Selecting a lead for an enzyme target requires either a detailed knowledge of the biochemistry of the pathological condition or using techniques such as computational (Chapter 5) and combinatorial chemistry (Chapter 6). One advantage of targeting enzymes is that an enzyme process that occurs in a pathogen may not occur in humans. This means that an inhibitor active in a pathogen should not inhibit the same process in humans.

Enzyme inhibitors (I) may have either a reversible or irreversible action. Reversible inhibitors tend to bind to an enzyme (E) by electrostatic bonds, hydrogen bonds and van der Waals' forces, and so tend to form an equilibrium system with the enzyme. A few reversible inhibitors bind by weak covalent bonds, but this is the exception rather than the rule. Irreversible inhibitors usually bind to an enzyme by strong covalent bonds. However, in both reversible and irreversible inhibition the inhibitor does not need to bind to the active site in order to prevent enzyme action.

Reversible: $E + I \rightleftharpoons E - I$ complex
Irreversible: $E + I \rightarrow E - I$ complex

7.3.1 Reversible inhibitors

These are inhibitors that form a dynamic equilibrium system with the enzyme. The inhibitory effects of reversible inhibitors are normally time dependent because the removal of unbound inhibitor from the vicinity of its site of action by natural processes will disturb this equilibrium to the left. As a result, more enzyme becomes available, which causes a decrease in the inhibition of the process catalysed by the enzyme. Consequently, reversible enzyme inhibitors will only be effective for a specific period of time.

Most reversible inhibitors may be further classified as being either **competitive, non-competitive** or **uncompetitive**. In **competitive inhibition** the inhibitor *usually* binds by a reversible process to the same active site of the enzyme as the substrate. Since the substrate and inhibitor compete for the same active site it follows that they will probably be structurally similar (Figure 7.3). This offers a rational approach to drug design in this area.

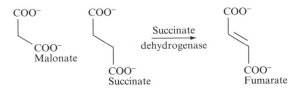

Figure 7.3 The similarity of the structures of malonate and succinate explains why malonate inhibits succinate dehydrogenase

Non-competitive inhibitors bind reversibly to an allosteric site (see Appendix 7) on the enzyme. In **pure** non-competitive inhibition, the binding of the inhibitor to the enzyme does not influence the binding of the substrate to the enzyme. However, this situation is uncommon, and the binding of the inhibitor usually causes conformational changes in the structure of the enzyme, which in turn affects the binding of the substrate to the enzyme. This is known as **mixed** non-competitive inhibition. The fact that the inhibitor does not bind to the active site of the enzyme means that the structure of the substrate cannot be used as the basis of designing new drugs that act in this manner to inhibit enzyme action.

Uncompetitive inhibitors are believed to form a complex with the enzyme–substrate complex. The formation of this complex prevents the substrate reacting to form its normal product(s).

7.3.2 Irreversible inhibition

Irreversible inhibitors may be classified for convenience as **active site directed inhibitors** and **suicide** or **irreversible mechanism based inhibitors (IMBIs)**. They bind to the enzyme by either strong non-covalent or strong covalent bonds. Inhibitors bound by strong non-covalent bonds will slowly dissociate, releasing the enzyme to carry out its normal function. However, whatever the type of binding, the enzyme will resume its normal function once the organism has synthesized a sufficient number of additional enzyme molecules to overcome the effect of the inhibitor.

Active site directed inhibitors are compounds that bind at or near to the active site of the enzyme. These inhibitors usually form strong covalent bonds with either the functional groups that are found at the active site or close to that site. Since these groups are usually nucleophiles, the incorporation of electrophilic groups in the structure of a substrate can be used to develop new inhibitors (Table 7.3). This approach may also be used to enhance the action of a known inhibitor. Most of the active site directed irreversible inhibitors in clinical use were not developed from a substrate. They were obtained or developed by other routes and only later was their mode of action discovered. For example, aspirin,

Table 7.3 Examples of the electrophilic groups used to produce active site directed inhibitors

Nucleophilic group of enzyme (E)	Electrophilic group	Product
$E-NH_2$	Anhydrides RCOOCOR	Amides RCONH–E
	Ketones $> C = O$	Imines $> C = N - E$
	Arenesulphonyl halides RSO_2X	Arenesulphonamides RSO_2NH-E
$E-COOH$	Epoxides $R-\!\!\triangle\!\!^{O}$	Hydroxyesters $RCH(OH)CH_2CO_2-E$
	α-Haloacetates $X-CH_2CO_2^-$	Half esters $^-O_2CCHCO_2-E$
$E-OH$	Phosphoryl halides $(RO)_2PO(X)$	Phosphates $(RO)_2OPO-E$
	Carbamates RNHCOOR	Carbamates RNHCOO–E
$E-SH$	α-Haloesters $X-CH_2CO_2R$	Sulphides $ROCOCH_2-S-E$
	α-Haloacetates $X-CH_2CO_2^-$	Sulphides $ROCOCH_2-S-E$
	Epoxides $R-\!\!\triangle\!\!^{O}$	Hydroxy sulphides $RCH(OH)CH_2-S-E$

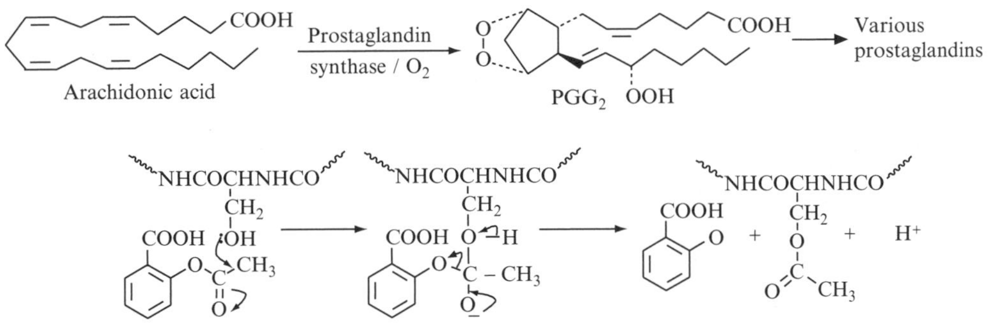

Figure 7.4 The biosynthesis of prostaglandins

first used clinically at the end of the 19th century as an antipyretic, is now believed to irreversibly inhibit prostaglandin synthase (cyclooxygenase), the enzyme that catalyses the conversion of arachidonic acid to PGG_2 (Appendix 8), which acts as a source for a number of other prostaglandins (Figure 7.4). Experimental evidence suggests that aspirin acts by acetylating serine hydroxy groups at the enzyme's active site, probably by a transesterification mechanism.

Suicide inhibitors, alternatively known as K_{cat} or irreversible mechanism based inhibitors (IMBIs), are irreversible inhibitors that are often analogues of the normal substrate of the enzyme. The inhibitor binds to the active site, where it is modified by the enzyme to produce a reactive group, which reacts irreversibly to form a stable inhibitor–enzyme complex. This subsequent reaction may or may not involve functional groups at the active site. This means that suicide inhibitors are likely to be specific in their action, since they can only be activated by a particular enzyme. This specificity means that drugs designed as suicide inhibitors could exhibit a lower degree of toxicity.

A wide variety of structures have been found to act as sources of the electrophilic groups of suicide inhibitors (Figure 7.5). These structures will only give rise to an electrophilic group if the compound containing the structure can act as a substrate for the enzyme. They often take the form of α,β unsaturated carbonyl compounds and imines formed by the reverse of a Michael addition at the active site of the enzyme.

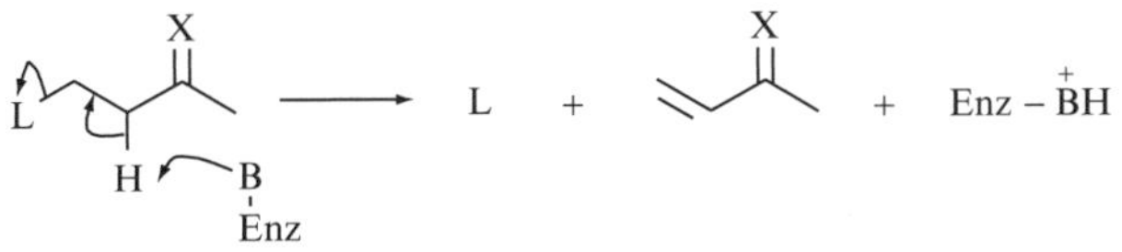

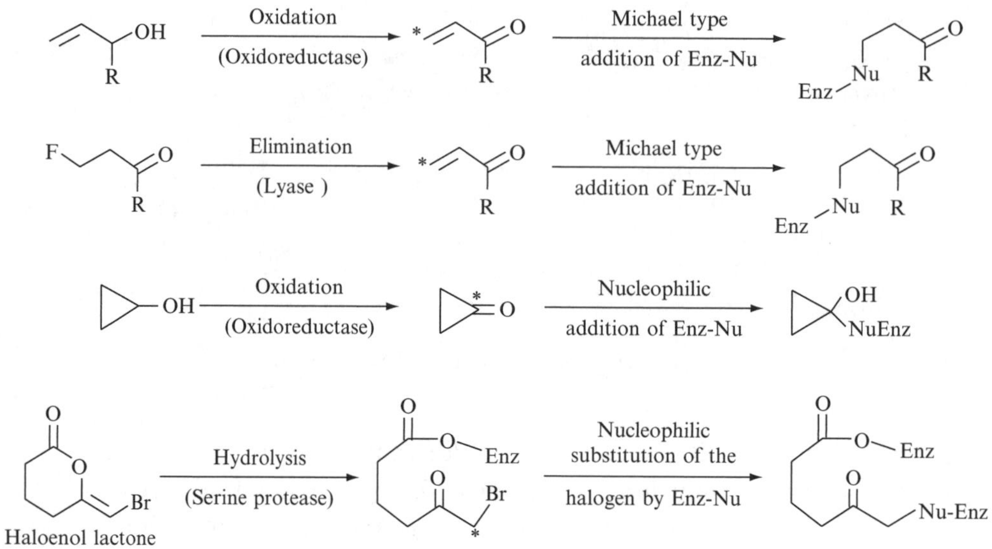

Figure 7.5 Examples of the reactions to enhance or form the electrophilic centres* of suicide inhibitors and their subsequent reaction with a nucleophile at the active site of the enzyme. The general structures used for the enzyme–inhibitor complexes are to illustrate the reactions; the enzyme ester groups may or may not be present in the final complex

The α,β unsaturated carbonyl compounds and imines formed in this manner react by a type of Michael addition with nucleophilic groups (Nu), such as the OH of serine residues, the SH of cysteine residues and the ω-NH$_2$ of lysine residues, frequently found at the active sites of enzymes.

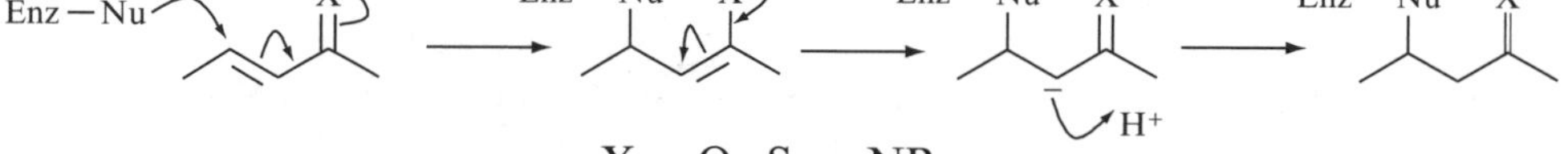

$$X = O, \text{ S or } NR$$

7.3.3 Transition state inhibitors

The substrate in an enzyme catalysed reaction is converted to the product through a series of transition state structures (Appendix 7). Although these transition state structures are transient, they bind to the active site of the enzyme and therefore must have structures that are compatible with the structure of the active site. Consequently, it has been proposed that *stable compounds* with structures similar to those of these transition state structures could bind to the active site of an enzyme and act as inhibitors for that enzyme. Compounds that fulfil this requirement are known as **transition state inhibitors**. They may act in either a reversible or irreversible manner.

The structures of transition states may be deduced using classical chemistry and mechanistic theory. These structures may also be visualized using computers (see Chapter 5). The resultant transition state structure and/or pictures may be used as the starting point for the design of a transition state inhibitor. For example, in the early 1950s it was observed that some rat liver tumours appeared to utilize more uracil in DNA formation than healthy liver. The first step in the biosynthesis of pyrimidines is the condensation of aspartic acid with carbamoyl phosphate to form N-carbamoyl aspartic acid, the reaction being catalysed by aspartate transcarbamoylase (Figure 7.6(a)). It has been proposed that the transition state for this conversion involves the simultaneous loss of phosphate with the attack of the nucleophilic amino group of the aspartic acid on the carbonyl group of the carbamoyl phosphate (Figure 7.6(b)). Consequently, the structure of the experimental anticancer drug, sodium N-phosphonoacetyl-L-aspartate (PALA, Figure 7.6(c)), was based on the structure of this transition state but without the amino group necessary for the next stage in the

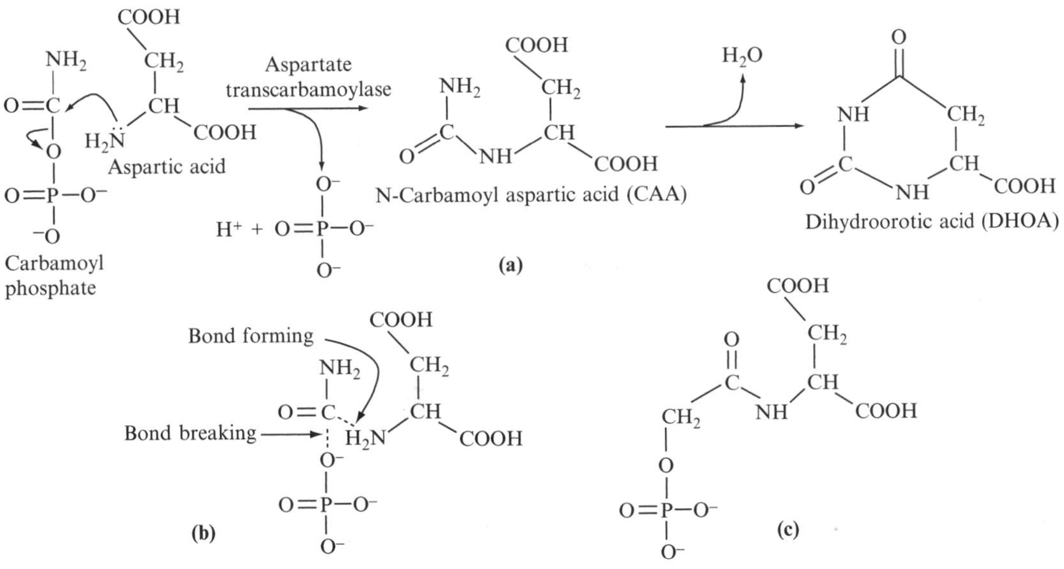

Figure 7.6 (a) The first step in the biosynthesis of pyrimidines. (b) The proposed transition state for the carbamoyl phosphate/aspartic acid stage in pyrimidine synthesis. (c) The structure of sodium N-phosphonoacetyl-L-aspartate (PALA)

synthesis, which is the conversion of N-carbamoyl aspartatic acid to dihydrooro-
tic acid. It was found that PALA bound 10^3 times more tightly to the enzyme than
the normal substrate, and was effective against some cancers in rats.

7.4 Drugs that target receptors

The binding of a drug to a receptor (Appendix 4) either inhibits the action of the
receptor or stimulates the receptor to give the physiological responses that are
characteristic of the action of the drug. Drugs that bind to a receptor and give a
similar response to that of the endogenous ligand are known as **agonists**,
whereas drugs that bind to a receptor but do not cause a response are termed
antagonists. Viruses, bacteria and toxins may also bind to the receptor sites of
specific tissues. This may cause unwanted pharmacological effects to occur.

7.4.1 Agonists

The response due to an agonist increases with increasing agonist concentration
until that response reaches a maximum (Figure 7.8(a)). At this point, further
increases in agonist concentration have no further effect on the response.

Agonists often have structures that are similar to that of the endogenous
ligand (Figure 7.7). Consequently, the normal starting point for the design of

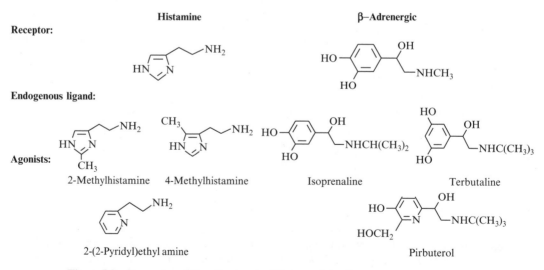

Figure 7.7 Examples of the structures of the agonists of some common receptors

new agonists is usually the structure of the endogenous ligand or its pharmaco-phore. This information is normally obtained from a study of the binding of the endogenous ligand to the receptor using X-ray crystallography, nuclear magnetic resonance (NMR) and computerized molecular modelling techniques. However, it is emphasized that many agonists have structures that are not directly similar to those of their endogenous ligands.

A common approach to designing new drugs that act on a receptor is to synthesize and investigate the activity of a series of compounds with similar structures to that of either compounds that are known to bind to the receptor, the endogenous ligand or the pharmacophore of the endogenous ligand (Table 7.4). This approach is an example of the use of SAR discussed in chapter 4. It is based on the assumption that a new agonist is more likely to be effective if its structure contains the same binding groups and bears some resemblance to the endogenous ligand.

The binding groups are not the only consideration when designing a drug to act at a receptor; the drug must also be of the correct size and shape to bind to and activate the receptor. Once again, the initial approach is to use the structure of the endogenous ligand or other active compounds as models. If sufficient data is available to construct a computer model of the receptor, the docking procedure (see section 5.5) may be used to check whether a lead or its analogues is likely to be able to bind to that receptor. Information concerning the best shape for a new agonist may also be obtained from a study of the conformations and configurations of a number of active analogues of the endogenous ligand.

7.4.2 Antagonists

Antagonists are ligands that inhibit the action of an agonist. Their are classified as either **competitive** or **non-competitive**. Competitive antagonists bind to the

Table 7.4 A series of compounds typical of that used in a search for a new agonist for the neurotransmitter acetylcholine. The activity is given in terms of the molar ratio needed to give the same degree of potency as acetylcholine

Structure	Activity		Structure	Activity	
	Cat blood pressure	Frog heart		Cat blood pressure	Frog heart
$CH_3COOCH_2CH_2\overset{+}{N}(CH_3)_3$ Acetylcholine	1	1	$CH_3COOCH_2CH_2\overset{+}{N}H(CH_3)_2$	50	50
$CH_3COOCH_2CH_2\overset{+}{N}H_2CH_3$	500	500	$CH_3COOCH_2CH_2\overset{+}{N}H_3$	2000	40 000
$CH_3COOCH_2CH_2\overset{+}{N}(C_2H_5)_3$	2000	10 000	$CH_3COOCH_2CH_2\overset{+}{P}(CH_3)_3$	13	12
$CH_3COOCH_2CH_2\overset{+}{S}(CH_3)_2$	50	96			

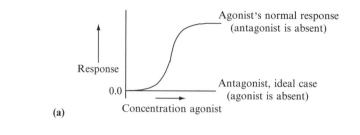

(a)

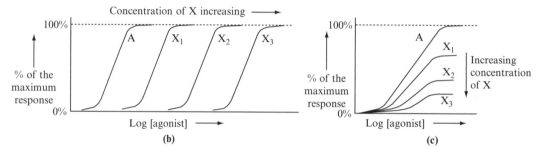

(b)   (c)

Figure 7.8 (a)   The effect of an ideal antagonist on the response of a receptor. (b) The effect of different concentrations of an ideal competitive antagonist X on the dose–response curve for an agonist A. (c) The effect of different concentrations of non-competitive antagonist on the dose–response curve of drug A. Key: The A plots are the dose–response curves for the agonist in the absence of the antgonist X. The X_1–X_3 plots are the dose–response curves for the agonist A in the presence of three different concentrations of the antagonist X .

same receptor as an agonist but do not cause a response (Figure 7.8(a)). As the concentration of the competitive antagonist increases, the response due to agonist decreases. However, increasing the concentration of the agonist will reverse this decrease (Figure 7.8(b)). It is believed that non-competitive antagonists bind irreversibly by strong bonds, such as covalent bonds, to allosteric sites on the receptor. This changes the conformation of the receptor site, which prevents the binding of the agonist to the receptor. In addition, increasing the concentration of the agonist does not restore the response of the receptor (Figure 7.8(c)).

The ideal starting point for the design of a new antagonist would be the structure of the receptor. However, it is often difficult to identify the receptor and also obtain the required structural and stereochemical information. Consequently, although it is not the ideal starting point, many developments start with the structure and stereochemistry of either the endogenous ligand or any other known agonists and antagonists for the receptor. Since antagonists exert a stronger affinity for the receptor than its natural agonist, the binding groups selected for the new drug are often groups that could form stronger bonds with the receptor. Furthermore, in order to bind to the receptor, the conformations and configuration of the new antagonist should be complementary to the structure of the receptor. If sufficient data is available, molecular modelling docking techniques (see section 5.5) can yield valuble insight into these aspects of the binding of the potential antagonist to the receptor.

7.4.3 Partial agonists

Partial agonists are compounds that act as both agonists and antagonists. They are believed to act as antagonists by preventing the endogenous ligand binding to the receptor but at the same time weakly activating the receptor. This is thought to cause a weak signal to be sent to the appropriate domain of the receptor. The net result of these opposing effects is that a much higher dose of the agonist is required to obtain the maximum response. Furthermore, this response is less than that of pure agonists with similar structures. Most drugs are partial agonists.

7.5 Drugs that target nucleic acids

Drugs that target DNA and RNA (see Chapter 1) either inhibit the synthesis of DNA and RNA or act on existing nucleic acid molecules. Those that inhibit the synthesis of nucleic acids usually act as antimetabolites and enzyme inhibitors. Those that act on existing nucleic acid molecules may for convenience by broadly classified as intercalating agents, alkylating agents and chain cleaving agents. In both cases, the net result is the prevention or slowing down of cell growth and division. Consequently, the discovery of new drugs that target existing DNA and RNA is a major line of approach for the development of new drugs for the treatment of cancer (see Appendix 10) and bacterial and other infections due to microorganisms.

7.5.1 Antimetabolites

Antimetabolites are compounds that block the normal metabolic pathways operating in cells. They act by either replacing an endogenous compound in the pathway by a compound whose incorporation into the system either results in a product that can no longer play any further part in the pathway or inhibits an enzyme in the metabolic pathway in the cell. Both these types of intervention inhibit the targeted metabolic pathway to a level that hopefully has a significant effect on the health of the patient.

The nature of the action of antimetabolites means that a rational starting point for the design of new drugs is the structure of the normal metabolites used by the cell (Table 7.5). Consequently, SAR studies based on the endogenous metabolite supported by combinatorial synthesis and molecular modelling offer logical routes to new lead compounds and ultimately new drugs.

Antimetabolites that are used to prevent the formation of DNA may be classified as **antifolates, purine antimetabolites** and **pyrimidine antimetabolites** (Table 7.5). Antifolates are believed to inhibit dihydrofolate reductase (DHFR). This enzyme is responsible for catalysing the conversion of dihydrofolic acid (DHF or FH$_2$) to tetrahydrofolic acid (THF or FH$_4$), which occurs in

Table 7.5 Examples of antimetabolites

Classification and endogenous metabolite	Examples of antimetabolite	Notes
Antifolates 	 Methotrexate Aminopeterin	Methotrexate and aminopterin are believed to inhibit dihydrofolate reductase by blocking the reduction of dihydrofolate to tetrahydrofolate, which is the cofactor in the synthesis of thymine and purines used in DNA synthesis.
Purine antimotabolites 	Methyl transfer from MeFH$_4$ 6-Mercaptopurine 6-Thioguanidine	6-Mercaptopurine acts as the precursor of 6-thioguanosine-5'-phosphate, which inhibits several of the biochemical pathways for the synthesis of purine nucleotides. 6-Thioguanine is converted into 6-thioinosine-5'-phosphate, which disrupts DNA synthesis.
Pyridine antimetabolites	 Fluorouracil Cytarabine	They are thought to act by inhibiting one or more of the enzymes required for DNA synthesis.

the biosynthesis of purines and pyrimidines (Figure 7.9). In addition, DHFR also catalyses the conversion of folic acid to DHF.

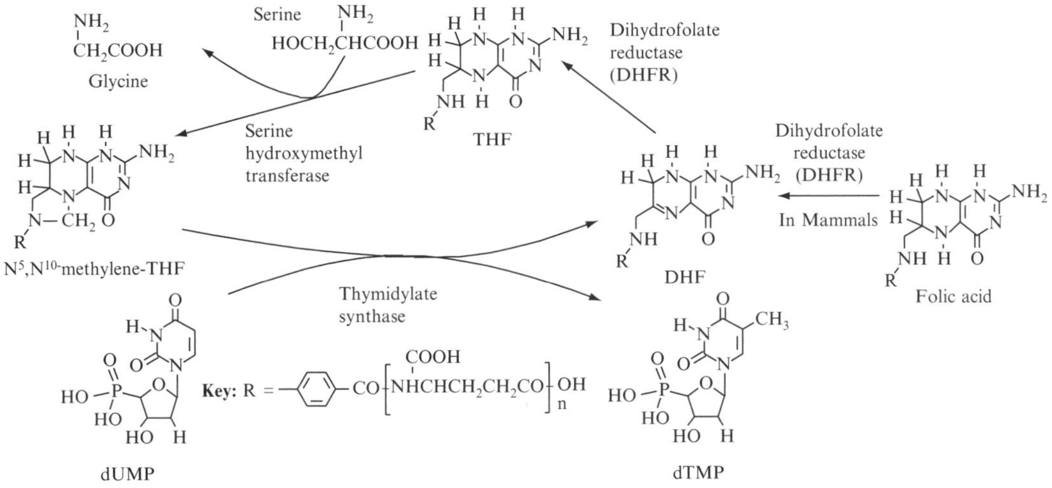

Figure 7.9 An outline of the synthesis of deoxythymidylate monophosphate (dTMP) from 2-deoxyuridylate monophosphate (dUMP). N^5, N^{10}-methylene-THF is the source of the methyl group in the conversion. Antifolates such as methotrexate inhibit DHFR

Purine antimetabolites are exogenous compounds, such as 6-mercaptopurine and 6-thioguanine, with structures based on the purine nucleus. They inhibit the synthesis of DNA and in some cases RNA by a number of different mechanisms. Pyrimidine antimetabolites have structures that closely resemble those of the endogenous pyrimidine bases. They usually act by inhibiting one or more of the enzymes that are required for DNA synthesis. For example, fluorouracil is metabolized by the same metabolic pathway as uracil to 5-fluoro-2'-deoxyuridyline monophosphate (FdUMP). FdUMP inhibits the enzyme thymidylate synthetase, which is responsible for the transfer of a methyl group from N^5, N^{10}-methylene-THF to the C5 atom of deoxyuridylate (dUMP) (Figure 7.9). The FdUMP binds to the enzyme but the presence of the unreactive C5-F bond in FdUMP blocks methylation of the FdUMP and as a result the formation of deoxythymidylate monophosphate (dTMP) and its subsequent incorporation into DNA (Figure 7.10). Fluorine was chosen to replace hydrogen at the C5 position because it is of a similar size to hydrogen (atomic radii: F, 0.13 nm, H, 0.12 nm). It was thought that this similarity in size would give a drug that would cause little steric disturbance to the biosynthetic pathway. In other words, the FdUMP would be the correct size and shape bind to the same active site of the enzyme as dUMP. Analogues containing larger halogen atoms do not have any appreciable activity because they are too large to bind effectively to the actve site of the enzyme.

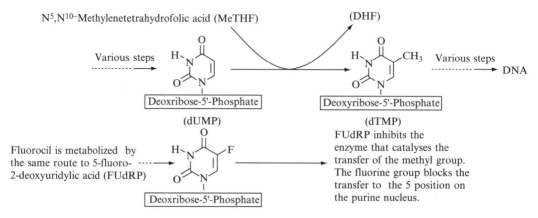

Figure 7.10   The intervention of fluorouracil in pyrimidine biosynthesis

7.5.2 Enzyme inhibitors

Enzyme inhibitors may inhibit the enzymes directly responsible for the formation of nucleic acids. For example, the topoisomerases, a group of enzymes that are responsible for the supercoiling, cleavage and rejoining of DNA, are inhibited by a number of compounds (Figure 7.11). This inhibition is believed to prevent DNA transcription, which ultimately leads to cell death, which explains the use of these drugs to treat cancer.

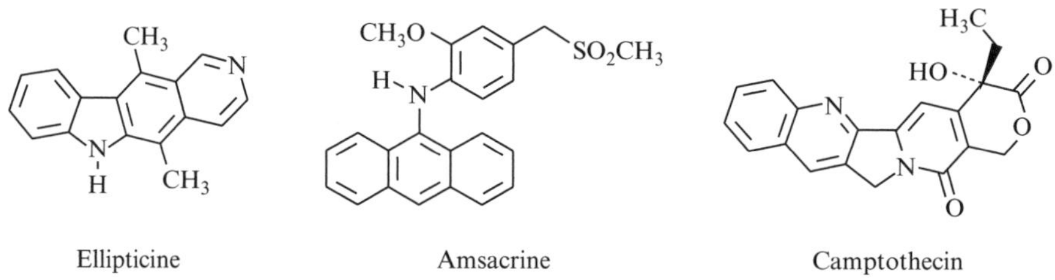

Ellipticine   Amsacrine   Camptothecin

Figure 7.11   Examples of topoisomerase inhibitors. Ellipticene acts by both intercalation and inhibition of topoisomerase II enzymes. It is active against nasopharyngeal carcinomas. Amsacrine is used to treat ovarian carcinomas, lymphomas and myelogenous leukaemias. Camptothecin is an antitumour agent

A wide range of compounds also inhibit a number of the enzyme systems that are involved in the biosynthesis of purines and pyrimidines in bacteria. For example, sulphonamide bacteriostatics inhibit dihydropteroate synthetase, which prevents the formation of folic acid in both humans and bacteria. However, although both mammals and bacteria synthesize their folic acid from PABA (Figure 7.12), mammals can also obtain it from their diet. In contrast, trimethoprim specifically inhibits bacterial DHF, which prevents the conversion of folic acid to DHF and DFH to THF (see Figures 7.9 and 7.12). Trimethoprim binds to bacterial DHFR but not human DHFR because of differences in the structures of these enzymes due to difference in species (Appendix 12). These observations led to the development of co-trimoxazole, a mixture of one part trimethoprim and five parts sulphamethoxazole, to treat bacterial infections

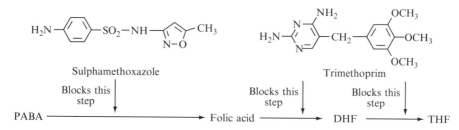

Sulphamethoxazole

Trimethoprim

Blocks this step | Blocks this step | Blocks this step |

PABA ⟶ Folic acid ⟶ DHF ⟶ THF

Figure 7.12 Sequential blocking using sulphamethoxazole and trimethoprim

7.5.3 Intercalation agents

Intercalating agents are compounds that insert themselves between the bases of the DNA helix (Figure 7.13(a)). The insertion causes the DNA helix to partially unwind at the site of the intercalated molecule. This inhibits transcription, which blocks the replication process of the cell. Although the mechanism of this inhibition is not known, inhibition of cell replication can lead to cell death and an improvement in the health of the patient.

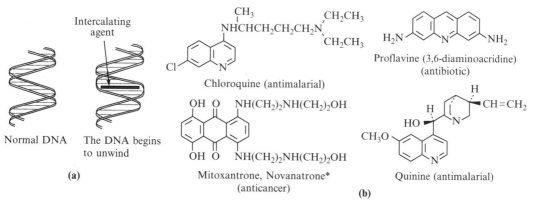

Figure 7.13 (a) A schematic representation of the action of intercalation agents. The horizontal dotted lines represent the complementary base pairs. The rings of these bases and the intercalating agent are on edge to the reader. (b) Examples of intercalating agents.[*] Trade name

The insertion of an intercalation agent appears to occur via either the minor or major grooves of DNA. Compounds that act as intercalating agents normally have structures that contain a flat fused aromatic or heteroaromatic ring system that can fit between the flat structures of the bases of the DNA (Figure 7.13(b)). These structures are believed to be held in place in the DNA by hydrogen bonds, van der Waals' forces and charge transfer bonds.

7.5.4 Alkylating agents

Alkylating agents are believed to bond to the nucleic acid chains in either the major or minor grooves. In DNA the alkylating agent frequently forms either **intrastrand** or **interstrand links**. Intrastrand cross linking agents form a bridge between two parts of the same chain. This has the effect of distorting the strand, which inhibits transcription. Interstrand cross links are formed between the two separate chains of the DNA, which has the effect of locking them together. This also inhibits transcription, which can ultimately lead to cell death. In both cases the nucleophilic nature of nucleic acids means that alkylating agents are usually either electrophiles or *in situ* give rise to electrophiles. Since the structures of DNA are relatively easy to model on a computer, the molecular modelling docking technique (see section 5.5) is a very useful tool for determining whether a compound is of a suitable size and shape to bind to a section of a nucleic acid. A wide range of different classes of compounds have been found to act as nucleic acid alkylating agents (Table 7.6). Their modes of action are not usually fully understood. However, a large amount of information is available concerning their structure–action relationships.

7.5.5 Antisense drugs

The concept of antisense compounds or sequence defined oligonucleotides (ONs) offers a new specific approach to designing drugs that target nucleic acids. The idea underlying this approach is that the antisense compound contains the sequence of bases complementary to those found in a short section of the target nucleic acid. The antisense compound binds to the target nucleic acid by hydrogen bonding between its the bases and the complementary bases of the target. This inhibits the normal function of the nucleic acid, which hopefully leads to the desired clinical response. Antisense compounds are able to bind to both RNA and DNA. In the latter case they form a triple helix.

Table 7.6 Some examples of the classes and compounds of anti-cancer agents that act by alkylation of nucleic acids. It is emphasized that this table only lists some of the classes of alkylating compound that are active against cancers

Class (based on)	Examples	Active against
Nitrogen mustard	Melphalan	Multiple myeloma, ovarian and breast carcinoma.
Triazeneimidazoles	Dacarbazine	Wide range including malignant lymphomas, malanomas and sarcomas.
Alkyl dimethanesulphonates $RO_2SOCH_2CH_2CH_2CH_2OSO_2R$	Busulphan	Granulocytic leukaemia.
Nitrosoureas –NHCON(NO)–	$ClCH_2CH_2NHCONCH_2CH_2Cl$ Carmustine	Active against cancers of the brain and cerebrospinal fluid.
Imidazotetrazinones	Temozolomide	Melanoma and brain tumours.
Platinum complexes	Carboplatin	Testicular and ovarian cancers.
Carbinolamines –NR– CHOH–	Trimenlamol	Ovarian cancer.

Antisense compounds were originally short lengths of nucleic acid chains that had base sequences that were complementary to those found in their target RNA. These compounds were found to be unsuitable as drugs because of poor binding to the target site and short half lives due to enzyme catalysed hydrolysis. At present, development is still in its early stages, but the concept has aroused considerable interest in the pharmaceutical industry. Development is currently taking three basic routes:

1. modification of the backbone to increase stability to hydrolysis (Figure 7.14(b));

2. changing the nature of the sugar residue (Figure 7.14(c)) and

3. modifying the nature of the substituent groups of the bases (Figure 7.14(d)).

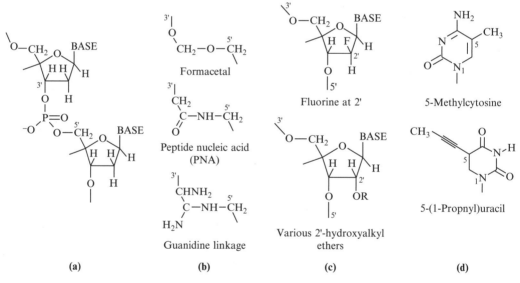

Figure 7.14   Development routes for antisense drugs. Examples of (a) a section of the backbone of a deoxyribonucleic chain, (b) backbone modifications, (c) sugar residue modifications and (d) base modifications

7.5.6 Chain cleaving agents

The interaction of chain cleaving agents with DNA results in the breaking of the nucleic acid into fragments. Currently, the main cleaving agents are the bleomycins and their analogues (Figure 7.15). These are a group of naturally

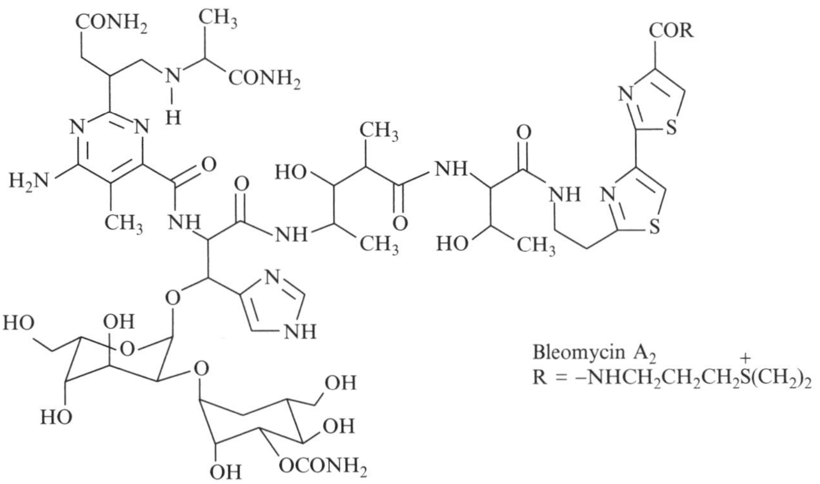

Figure 7.15 The bleomycins. The drug bleomycin sulphate is a mixture of a number of bleomycins

occuring glycoproteins that exhibit antitumour activity. Their action is not understood, but the nucleic acid fragments produced cannot be rejoined by DNA ligases. Unfortunately, they exhibit a number of unwanted side effects. However, other classes of drug are in the development stage.

7.6 Antiviral drugs

It has been found that viruses (Appendix 10) utilize a number of virus specific enzymes during replication. These enzymes and the processes they control are significantly different from those of the host cell to make a useful target for medicinal chemists. Consequently, antiviral drugs usually act by either inhibiting viral nucleic acid synthesis, inhibit attachment to and penetration of the host cell or inhibit viral protein synthesis.

7.6.1 Nucleic acid synthesis inhibitors

These drugs usually act by inhibiting the polymerases or reverse transcriptases required for nucleic acid synthesis. They are usually analogues of the purine and pyrimidine bases found in the nucleic acids (Figure 7.16). Their general mode of action often involves conversion to the corresponding triphosphate by the host

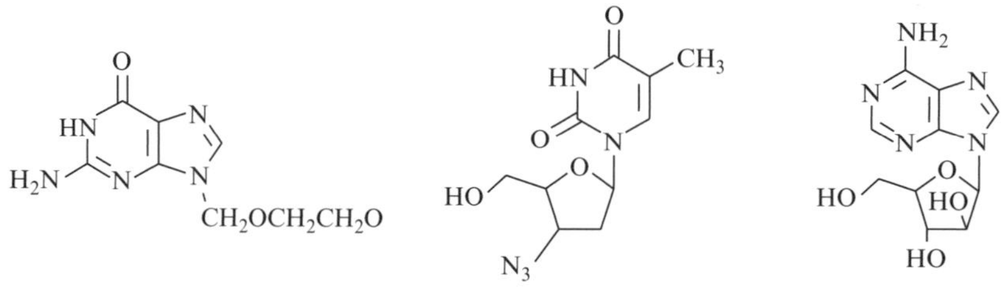

Acyclovir   Zidovudine (AZT)   Vidarabine

Figure 7.16 Examples of viral nucleic acid synthesis inhibitors that form triphosphate drug derivatives *in situ*

cell's cellular kinases. This conversion may also involve specific viral enzymes in the initial monophosphorylation step. These triphosphate drug derivatives are incorporated into the nucleic acid chain, where they terminate its formation. Termination occurs because the drug residues do not have a 3′ hydroxy group necessary for the phosphate ester formation, required for further growth of the nucleic acid chain. This effectively inhibits the polymerases and transcriptases that catalyse the growth of the nucleic acid. In addition, these drugs also inhibit other enzymes involved in the nucleic acid chain formation.

7.6.2 Host cell penetration inhibitors

The principal drugs that act in this manner are amantadine and rimantadine (Figure 7.17). Amantadine hydrochloride is effective against influenza A virus but is not effective against the influenza B virus. It is believed to acts by blocking an ion channel in the virus membrane formed by the viral protein M_2. This is believed to inhibit the disassembly of the core of the virion and its penetration of the host. However, its use can result in depression, dizziness, insomnia and gastrointestinal disturbances amongst other unwanted side effects. Rimantadine hydrochloride is an analogue of amantadine hydrochloride that exhibits significantly fewer CNS side effects.

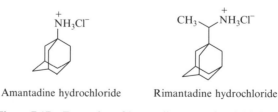

Amantadine hydrochloride   Rimantadine hydrochloride

Figure 7.17 Examples of host cell penetration inhibitors

7.6.3 Inhibitors of viral protein synthesis

The principal compounds that act as inhibitors of viral protein synthesis are the **interferons**. These compounds are members of a naturally occurring family of glycoprotein hormones (RMM 20 000–160 000), which are produced by nearly all types of eukaryotic cell. Three general classes of interferons are known to occur naturally in mammals, namely; the α-interferons produced by leucocytes, β-interferons produced by fibroblasts and γ-interferons produced by T lymphocytes. They form part of the human immune system. It is believed that the presence of virons and pathogens in the body switches on the mRNA that stimulates the production and release of interferons. These interferons are thought to stimulate the production of proteins that inhibit the synthesis of viral mRNA and viral proteins. α-Interferons also enhance the activity of T killer cells.

The formation and release of interferon by viral and other pathological stimulation has resulted in a search for chemical inducers of endogenous interferon. Administration of a wide range of compounds has resulted in induction of interferon production. However, no clinically useful compounds have been found for humans, although tilorone is effective in inducing interferon in mice.

Tilorone

7.7 Questions

(1) Describe the main differences between each of the following:
  (a) fungicidal and fungistatic drugs;
  (b) agonist and antagonist and
  (c) eukaryotic and prokaryotic cells.

(2) What are ionophores? How do they act?

(3) Suggest reasons for bacterial resistance to β-lactam drugs.

(4) Describe the main features of competitive, non-competitive and irreversible inhibition of enzymes.

(*continues overleaf*)

(*continued*)

  (5) Explain the meaning of the term 'suicide inhibitor'.

  (6) Explain how the transition state of a reaction can be used to design an enzyme inhibitor.

  (7) Distinguish between competitive and noncompetitive antagonists.

  (8) Explain the meaning of the term antimetabolite. Outline, in general terms, the mode of action of antimetabolite drugs.

  (9) Draw the general structure of nitrogen mustards. How do these drugs inhibit the transcription of DNA?

(10) What are antisense drugs? How do they inhibit nucleic acids?

(11) Outline, using suitable examples, the general modes of action of antiviral drugs.

8 Pharmacokinetics

8.1 Introduction to pharmacokinetics

The action of a drug is initially dependent on it reaching its site of action in sufficient concentration for a long enough period of time for a significant pharmacological response to occur. The concentration range over which the drug is effective is referred to as its therapeutic window (see section 2.6). The relationship of this concentration to the dose administered is not simple (Figure 8.2). Once a drug is absorbed into the body it must find its way to its site of action. In the course of this transportation some of the drug will be metabolized (see Chapter 9) and some will be irreversibly excreted by the liver and/or kidneys and/or lungs. The **irreversible** processes by which a drug is prevented from reaching its site of action are collectively referred to as **elimination**. However, uptake into the tissues is not regarded as an elimination process since it is usually reversible, the drug returning to the general circulation system (systemic circulation) in the course of time (Figure 8.1).

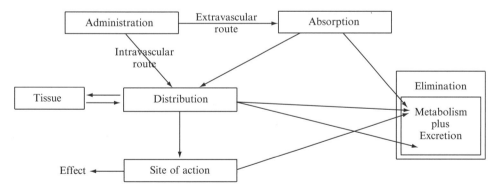

Figure 8.1 The general stages and their relationships in the life cycle of a drug after administration

Fundamentals of Medicinal Chemistry, Edited by Gareth Thomas
© 2003 John Wiley & Sons, Ltd
ISBN 0 470 84306 3 (Hbk), ISBN 0 470 84307 1 (pbk)

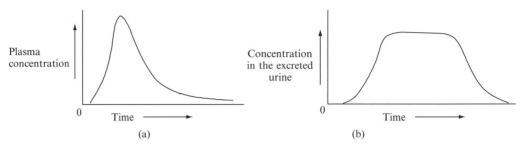

Figure 8.2 Typical variations in the concentration of a drug with time in samples of (a) plasma and (b) urine after the administration of a single oral dose of the drug at time zero. In both cases the precise shape of the graph will depend on the drug being studied

The process of elimination means that it is important to have a method of monitoring the concentration of a drug in contact with its site of action. Since the precise site of action is often unknown the concentration of the drug is usually monitored by following the concentration of the drug in the plasma and other suitable body fluids (Figure 8.2). These measurements are statistically correlated with the effects of the drug on humans and, where this data is difficult to obtain, animals. However, the results of these animal experiments have been extrapolated to humans with varying degrees of success.

8.1.1 General classification of pharmacokinetic properties

The pharmacokinetic properties (ADME, see section 2.7.1) of a drug are specified in terms of measurable parameters such as plasma concentration, biological half-life and rate constants. The methods used to calculate these parameters are independent of the method of administration, although the values obtained will depend on the administrative route (see section 2.6). For example, intravascular routes will not normally give values for absorption parameters. However, intravascular routes do give higher concentrations of the drug in the general circulatory system (**systemic circulatory system**).

8.2 Pharmacokinetics and drug design

A study of the pharmacokinetic properties of a compound indicates which properties need to be modified in order to produce a more effective analogue. Consider, for example, a drug that is not suitable for development because it has too short a duration of action. The logical way forward is to determine the likely structural cause of this rapid elimination and then test analogues that either do not contain this structural function or have structures where it is sterically hindered. If, for example, the drug is rapidly metabolized by esterases in the plasma, compounds that are more stable to these enzymes would be tested. Alternatively, the drug may be poorly absorbed because it is very water soluble, in which case the approach is to produce and test less water soluble analogues. Pharmacokinetics may be used to provide the information required to design dosage regimens (section 2.6). It has been particularly useful in determining drug dosages for patients with damaged organs. It is also used to obtain information concerning the effect of drug metabolites in humans and other mammals.

8.3 Pharmacokinetic models

The accurate assessment of the results of a pharmacokinetic investigation requires the use of mathematical methods. In order to apply these methods to the behaviour of a drug, in what is a complex biological system it is necessary to use so called **model** systems. The commonly used **compartmental model** visualizes a biological system as a series of interconnected compartments (Figure 8.3). It allows the biological relationships between these compartments to be expressed in the form of mathematical equations. In all compartmental models, a compartment is defined as a group of tissues that have a similar blood flow and drug affinity. It is not necessarily a defined anatomical region in the body; however, all compartmental models systems assume that:

1. the compartments communicate with each other by reversible processes,

2. rate constants are used as a measure of the rate of entry and exit of a drug from a compartment,

3. the distribution of a drug within a compartment is rapid and homogeneous and

4. each drug molecule has an equal chance of leaving a compartment.

Compartmental models are normally based on a central compartment, which represents the plasma and the highly perfused tissues (Figure 8.3). Elimination (see section 2.7.1) of a drug is assumed to occur only from this compartment since the processes associated with elimination occur mainly in the plasma and the highly perfused tissues of the liver and kidney. Other compartments are connected to the central compartment as required by the nature of the investigation.

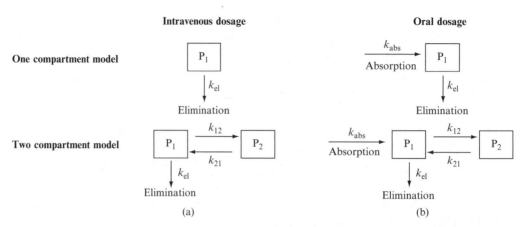

Figure 8.3 Compartmental models in which a drug is administered (a) by intravenous injection and (b) orally. The rate constant for the appropriate movement of the drug is k subscript. P_1 is the plasma and highly perfused tissue compartment, which is the central compartment in all compartmental models. It is the first destination of a drug

The simplest model is the one compartmental model, in which the compartment represents the circulatory system and all the tissues perfused by the drug (Figure 8.3). Other types of model are in use but unless stated otherwise all discussions in this text will be based on a one compartment model.

The information obtained using pharmacokinetic models has a wide variety of uses such as correlating drug doses with pharmacological and toxic responses and determining an optimum dose level for an individual. However, as these models are based on a simplification of what is a very complex system it is necessary to treat the results of these analyses with some degree of caution until the model has been rigorously tested.

8.4 Intravascular administration

The main methods of intravascular administration are intravenous (IV) injection and infusion. When a single dose of a drug is administered to a patient by intravenous injection, the dose is usually referred to as an **IV bolus**. Intravascular administration places the drug directly in the patient's circulatory system, which bypasses the body's natural barriers to drug absorption. Once it enters the circulatory system the drug is rapidly distributed to most tissues since a dynamic equilibrium is speedily reached between the drug in the blood and the tissue. This means that a fast IV bolus injection will almost immediately give a high initial concentration of the drug in the circulatory system but this will immediately start to fall because of elimination processes (Figure 8.4(a)). However, the plasma concentration of a drug administered by intravenous infusion will increase with time until the rate of infusion is equal to the rate of elimination (Figure 8.4(b)). At this point the drug plasma concentration remains constant until infusion is stopped whereupon it falls.

8.4.1 Intravenous injection (IV bolus)

The administration of a drug by a rapid intravenous injection places the drug in the circulatory system where it is distributed (see section 2.7.1) to all the accessible body compartments and tissues. The one compartment model (Figure 8.3(a)) of drug distribution assumes that the administration and distribution of the drug in the plasma and associated tissues is instantaneous. This does not happen in practice and is one of the possible sources of error when using this model to analyse experimental pharmacokinetic data.

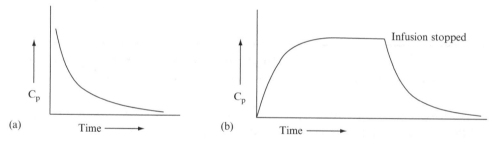

Figure 8.4 The variation of the concentration of a drug in the plasma (C_p) with time when administered by (a) a rapid single intravenous injection and (b) intravenous infusion. With rapid intravenous injections the graph does not show the time taken to carry out the injection; it is normally taken as being spontaneous. In these cases the curve starts at the point where the first plasma concentration measurements were taken

Once in the circulatory system the concentration of the drug begins to decline (Figure 8.4(a)). This decline, which is due to elimination processes (see section 2.7.1), is normally recorded by plotting a graph of the plasma concentration of the drug against time. These graphs are usually close to being exponential curves (Figure 8.4(a)), that is, elimination normally exhibits **first order kinetics**. This observation enables medicinal chemists to describe these elimination processes to an acceptable degree of accuracy by the mathematical equations used for **first order kinetics**, that is:

$$\text{rate of elimination} = k_{el} C \tag{8.1}$$

and

$$C = C_0 e^{-k_{el} t} \tag{8.2}$$

where C_0 is the plasma concentration of the drug in the body at a time $t = 0$, that is, the concentration immediately following bolus injection, C is the plasma concentration of the drug in the body at a time t, t is the lapsed time between the administration and the measurement and k_{el} is the rate constant for the irreversible elimination of the drug.

The plasma concentration C of a drug in the system is related to the total amount of the drug in the system D by the relationship:

$$C = D/V_d \tag{8.3}$$

where V_d is the apparent volume of distribution. The value of V_d is a measure of the total volume of the body perfused by the drug. It is an apparent volume because it is the volume of plasma that is **equivalent** to the total volume of the body readily perfused by the drug. It is not the volume of the tissue and the circulatory system actually perfused by the drug. This means that the values of V_d for a drug can be considerably higher than the volume of the blood in the circulatory system which is usually about 5 litres for a 70 kg person. Values of V_d are usually recorded in terms of litres per kilogram (Table 8.1), which gives a value of 0.071 (litres kg^{-1}) for a 70 kg person. A value of less than 0.071 for V_d indicates that the drug is probably distributed mainly within the circulatory system, whilst values greater than 0.071 indicate that the drug is distributed in both the circulatory system and specific tissues.

The value of V_d may be calculated by substituting the values for the dose D_0 administered and C_0, the plasma concentration at time $t = 0$, in equation (8.3). However, it is not possible to accurately measure the concentration of the drug in the system at the time $t = 0$ because of the time taken to administer a drug and for it to achieve a homogeneous distribution throughout the system. Consequently, a theoretical value of C_0 obtained by extrapolation of a plot of drug plasma concentration C_p against time (Figure 8.5) is normally used to calculate V_d.

Table 8.1 The values of V_d and $t_{1/2}$ for some common drugs (various sources)

Drug	V_d (litres kg^{-1})	$t_{1/2}$ (hours)	Drug	V_d (litres kg^{-1})	$t_{1/2}$ (hours)
Aspirin	0.1–0.2	0.28	Ibuprofen	0.14	2
Ampicillin	0.3	1–2	Propranolol	3.9	2–6
Cimetidine	2.1	1–3	Morphine	3.0–5.0	2–3
Chlorpromazine	20	15–30	Warfarin	0.15	42
Diazepam	1.0	48			

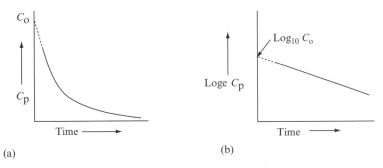

Figure 8.5 Determination of C_o by extrapolation of the plots of (a) the C_p against t curve and (b) log C_p against time for the changes in plasma concentration of a drug with time

The rate of elimination is an important characteristic of a drug. Too rapid an elimination necessitates frequent repeated administration of the drug if its concentration is to reach its therapeutic window. Conversely, too slow an elimination could result in the accumulation of the drug in the patient, which might give an increased risk of toxic effects. Most drug eliminations follow **first order kinetics** (equations (8.1) and (8.2)), no matter how the drug is administered, but there are some notable exceptions, such as ethanol which exhibits zero order kinetics where:

$$\text{rate} = k \text{ and } C = C_o - kt. \tag{8.4}$$

However, the order of elimination processes may change depending on the biological situation, for example, drug concentration increasing to a level that saturates the elimination processes, in which case first order eliminations processes will change to zero order.

The time taken for the concentration of a drug to fall to half its original value is known as its **biological half-life** ($t_{1/2}$). For eliminations that follow **first order kinetics** it may be shown that:

$$t_{1/2} = 0.693/k_{el} \tag{8.5}$$

In other words, for elimination processes that follow first order kinetics $t_{1/2}$ is a constant, characteristic of the drug and the biological system. Consequently, for drugs that exhibit **first order elimination kinetics** both and k_{el} and $t_{1/2}$ are used as indicators of the rate of elimination of a drug from the system. Half-lives are normally quoted in the literature and k_{el} values are calculated as required using equation (8.5).

For **first order** elimination processes the values of k_{el} and $t_{1/2}$ may be calculated from the experimental data using a logarithmic form of equation (8.2), that is for natural logarithms:

$$\ln C_p = \ln C_0 - k_{el}t \qquad (8.6)$$

and for logarithms to base 10:

$$\log_{10} C_p = \log_{10} C_0 - \frac{k_{el}t}{2.303} \qquad (8.7)$$

Both these equations give straight line plots (Figure 8.6) and so it is possible to obtain a value of k_{el} by measuring the slope of the graph provided the experimental data gives a reasonable straight line. The $t_{1/2}$ value may also be calculated from these graphs. However, it is advisable to take an average of several measurements of $t_{1/2}$ made from different initial values of C_p in order to obtain an accurate $t_{1/2}$ value.

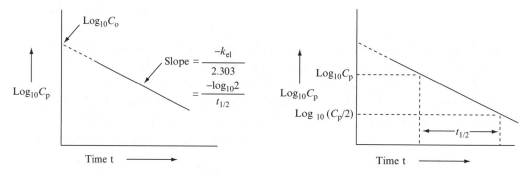

Figure 8.6   Determination of the values of $t_{1/2}$ and k_{el} from logarithmic plots of plasma concentration against time. The logarithm plot for logs to base ten is shown but the natural logarithmic plot would be similar except the slope would now be equal to k_{el}

Half-life and k_{el} values may be used to put the comparison of the pharmacological effect of a lead with its analogues on a numerical basis. This could provide an indication of the best course of action to take for the successful development of a useful drug. For example, if a lead has a short duration of action, analogues with larger $t_{1/2}$ and smaller k_{el} values than those of the lead are more likely to give the required pharmacological effect. Similarly, if the lead is too toxic, analogues with smaller $t_{1/2}$ and larger k_{el} values need to be developed. It is emphasized that $t_{1/2}$ and k_{el} data are not infallible and should not be considered in isolation.

8.4.2   Clearance and its significance

Clearance (CL) is defined as the **volume** of blood in a specified region of the body that is cleared of a drug in **unit time**. It is the parameter that relates the rate of elimination of a drug from a defined region of the body to the plasma concentration of that drug. For example, the total clearance (Cl_T), that is, the volume of blood in the whole body cleared of a drug in unit time, is related to the rate of elimination by the equation:

$$\text{rate of elimination of a drug from the whole body} = Cl_T C_p \qquad (8.8)$$

The clearance of a drug from a specific region of the body is the sum of all the clearances of all the contributing processes in that region. For example, hepatic clearance (Cl_H) is the sum of the clearances due to metabolism (Cl_M) and excretion (Cl_{Bile}) in the liver, that is:

$$Cl_H = Cl_M + Cl_{Bile} \qquad (8.9)$$

However, it is emphasized that clearance is an artificial concept as it is not possible for a drug to be removed from only one part of the total volume of the blood in the body or organ.

For elimination processes exhibiting **first order kinetics** it can be shown that clearance is related to V_d, k_{el} and $t_{1/2}$ by the mathematical expressions:

$$Cl_T = k_{el} V_d \qquad (8.10)$$

and

$$Cl_T = V_d \frac{0.693}{t_{1/2}} \qquad (8.11)$$

Since both $t_{1/2}$ and k_{el} are constant for elimination processes **following first order kinetics**, Cl will also be constant. However, should the order of the elimination change due to a change in the biological situation, such as the drug concentration increasing to the point where it saturates the metabolic elimination pathways, then clearance may not be constant.

For an IV bolus, which places the drug directly in the circulatory system, total clearance (Cl_T) of the drug from the body can also be determined from the plots of C_p against t. The area under the curve (AUC) represents the total amount of the drug that reaches the circulatory system in time t. It is related to the dose administered by the relationship:

$$\text{dose} = Cl_T \cdot \text{AUC} \qquad (8.12)$$

This relationship holds true regardless of the way in which a single dose of the drug is administered. However, for enteral routes the dose is the amount absorbed (see section 2.6), not the dose administered. The relationship (8.12) may also be used to calculate the clearance that occurs in a specific time by simply measuring the AUC for that time.

Clearance will vary with body weight and so for comparison purposes values are normally quoted per kilogram of body weight (Table 8.2). It also varies with the degree of protein binding. A large proportion of a drug with a high degree of protein binding will exhibit a lower clearance value, since it will not be so readily available for elimination as a drug with a lower degree of protein binding.

Table 8.2 Clearance values of some drugs

Drug	Clearance ($cm^3\ min^{-1}\ kg^{-1}$)	Drug	Clearance ($cm^3\ min^{-1}\ kg^{-1}$)
Atropine	8	Bumetamide	3
Bupivacaine	8	Caffeine	1–2
Disopyramide	0.5–2 (dose dependent)	Ethambutol	9
Mepivacaine	5	Pentobarbitone	0.3–0.5
Ranitidine	about 10	Vancomycin	about 1

All drugs are carried to their site of action by the blood. The route normally requires the drug to pass through several organs, where some of the drug may be lost by elimination. This loss is known as *extraction*. The proportion of the drug removed by a single transit of the total dose of the drug through the organ is defined as:

$$E = \frac{C_{in} - C_{out}}{C_{in}} \quad (8.13)$$

where E is known as the extraction ratio. The extraction ratio has no units. Its values range from zero to unity. A value of 0.4 means that 40 per cent of the drug is irreversibly removed as it passes through the organ. The clearance of the organ is related to the rate of blood flow by the relationship:

$$Cl = QE \quad (8.14)$$

where Q (volume per unit time) is the rate of blood flow. Since the liver is a major site of metabolism and excretion, the hepatic extraction values (E_H) of many drugs have been determined (Table 8.3). Leads where $E_H \sim 1$ will seldom reach the general circulatory system in sufficient quantity to be therapeutically effective.

Clearance is a more useful concept in pharmacokinetics than either $t_{1/2}$ or k_{el}. It enables blood flow rate, which controls the rate at which a drug is delivered to

Table 8.3   The hepatic extraction values of some drugs

Drug E_H value < 0.3 (low)	Drug E_H value 0.3–0.7	Drug E_H value > 0.7 (high)
Antripyrine	Aspirin	Cocaine
Diazepam	Codeine	Lignocaine
Nitrazepam	Nifedipine	Nicotine
Warfarin	Nortriptyline	Propranolol

a specific region of the body, to be taken into account when assessing the pharmacokinetic behaviour of the drug in that region of the body (see section 8.5). Clearance values enable the medicinal chemist to compare the effect of structural changes on drug behaviour and as a result decide which analogues might yield drugs with the desired pharmacokinetic properties. Extraction ratios can also be used to link the required desirable characteristics of a potential new drug with the chemical structures of the analogues of a lead. Their use can lead to the avoidance of the loss of a potential drug by indicating the most effective dosage form.

8.4.3   Intravenous infusion

In intravenous infusion, the drug is infused into the vein at a steady rate. Initially, the plasma concentration of the drug increases as the amount of the infused drug exceeds the amount of the drug being eliminated (Figure 8.7). However, as the concentration of the drug in the plasma increases, the rate of elimination also increases, until the rate of infusion is equal to the rate of elimination, at which point the concentration of the drug in the plasma remains constant. As long as the infusion rate is kept constant, the drug plasma concentration will remain at this steady state level (C_{ss}). When infusion is stopped the drug

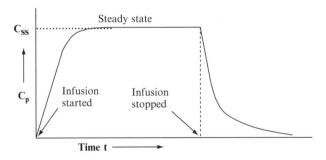

Figure 8.7   Plasma concentration changes with time in intravenous infusion

plasma concentration will fall, usually in an exponential curve, because the biological situation is now the same as if a dose of the drug had been given at that time by intravenous IV bolus injection (section 8.4.1).

The rate of change of the plasma concentration during intravenous infusion may be described by the relationship:

rate of change of plasma concentration $=$ rate of infusion $-$ rate of elimination (8.15)

Since the rate of infusion is normally maintained at a constant value, infusion will usually follow zero order kinetics (Equation (8.4)). Therefore, assuming that elimination processes exhibit first order kinetics, it follows that:

$$dC_p/dt = k_0 - k_{el}C_p \qquad (8.16)$$

where k_0 is the rate constant for the infusion. Initially the rate of infusion is greater than the rate of elimination, but at the the steady state the rate of elimination is equal to the rate of infusion and so the plasma concentration does not change.

$$\text{Consequently,} \ \ dC_p/dt = 0 \text{ and } k_{el}C_p = k_0 \qquad (8.17)$$

$$\text{but at the steady state } C_{ss} = C_p \qquad (8.18)$$

$$\text{and so } C_{ss} = \frac{k_0}{k_{el}} \qquad (8.19)$$

substituting for k_{el} from Equation (8.9) in Equation (8.19) gives:

$$C_{ss} = \frac{k_0 V_d}{Cl_T} = \frac{k_0^*}{Cl_T} \qquad (8.20)$$

where k_0^* is the amount of drug infused per unit time. Equations (8.19) and (8.20) can be used to calculate the rate of infusion required to achieve a specific steady state plasma concentration. These equations are independent of time and so an increase in the rate of infusion and a subsequent increase in the value of k_0 will not result in a reduction of the time taken to reach a specific value of C_{ss}. It will simply increase the value of C_{ss}, as the rate of elimination and hence k_{el} will remain constant. Consequently, too high a rate of infusion could increase the steady state plasma concentration of the drug to a value above the top limit of the therapeutic window for the drug, which in turn would increase the chances of a toxic response from the patient.

The time (t) taken to reach a specific value of C_p in the initial part of the infusion before the plasma concentration reaches the steady state concentration

(C_{ss}) may be calculated using Equation (8.21). This equation, which is derived from Equation (8.16) is based on the asumption that the initial stage of infusion follows first order kinetics.

$$t = -t_{1/2}1.44 \ \ln(1 - C_p/C_{ss}) \qquad (8.21)$$

At the steady state $C_p = C_{ss}$ and so the time taken to reach C_{ss} can be calculated by substituting $C_p/C_{ss} = 1$ in Equation (8.21). This time is dependent on the half-life value: the shorter the half-life the sooner the C_{ss} plateau is reached. Equation (8.21) also allows one to calculate the time taken to reach the effective plasma concentration, which is normally taken as being 90% of the C_{ss} value. In this case $C_p/C_{ss} = 0.9$. To reduce the time required to obtain an effective therapeutic plasma concentration, a single IV bolus injection may be given in conjunction with an IV infusion. As a result, the C_{ss} drug plasma concentration is reached almost immediately. However, once the drug enters the bloodstream it undergoes elimination, no matter what its original source, IV bolus or infusion. This elimination is compensated for by a build-up in the drug concentration from the intravenous infusion (Figure 8.8). At any time t the total concentration of the drug in the system is the sum of the drug from the IV bolus and the infusion. Its value is equal to the steady state concentration C_{ss} of the drug. The net result is that the patient almost immediately receives an almost constant effective therapeutic dose of the drug.

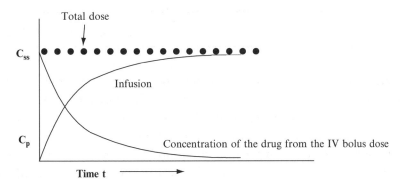

Figure 8.8   The effect of a single IV bolus on the plasma concentration of a drug administered by IV infusion

8.5 Extravascular administration

The most common form of enteral dosage form is oral administration. Consequently, this section will mainly be concerned with the pharmacokinetics of orally administered drugs. Most orally administered drugs are absorbed through the membranes of the GI tract. The rate of absorption will depend mainly on the rate of dissolution of the dosage form, that is, the rate at which the drug solid dosage forms passes into solution, the pH of the medium containing the drug (see Section 2.7.1), the lipid–aqueous medium partition coefficient of the drug and the surface area of the absorbing region of the GI tract.

Drugs absorbed from the GI tract must pass through the GI tract membrane, liver and other organs in order to reach the general circulation system. A fraction of the drug will be lost by metabolism and excretion as it follows this route to the circulatory system. These losses are referred to as the **first pass effect** or **first pass metabolism**. Since the main areas of excretion and metabolism in the systematic circulatory system are the enzyme-rich liver and lungs, the term is usually taken to refer to the elimination of a drug by these two organs. However, since the liver is the first organ the drug passes through after absorption from the GI tract and it is also the principal area of metabolism, the effect of the lungs is often ignored, and the term first pass metabolism is frequently used as though it involved only the liver.

The physiology of drug absorption from the GI tract has a direct effect on the **bioavailability** (F) of a drug. Bioavailability is defined as the fraction of the dose of a drug that enters the general circulatory system, that is:

$$F = \frac{\text{amount of drug that enters the general circulatory system}}{\text{dose administered}} \quad (8.22)$$

Since the area under the plasma concentration–time curve (AUC) for a drug is a measure of the total amount of a drug reaching the general circulatory system, the bioavailability of a drug may also be defined in terms of the AUC as:

$$F = \text{AUC/dose} \quad (8.23)$$

If all the dose of a drug reached the circulatory system, the bioavailability as defined by Equation (8.22) would have a value of unity 1. Therefore, if E is the extraction for first pass metabolism,

$$F = 1 - E \quad (8.24)$$

and so, for orally administered drugs, Equation (8.24) approximates to:

$$F = 1 - E_H \quad (8.25)$$

where E_H is the hepatic extraction ratio. Therefore, leads with high hepatic extraction values ($E_H{\sim}1$) will seldom reach the general circulatory system in sufficient quantity to be therapeutically effective if administered orally.

Bioavailability studies using animals are used to compare the efficiency of the delivery of the dosage forms of a drug to the general circulatory system as well as the efficiency of the route of administration for both licensed drugs and new drugs under development. Two useful measurements are **relative** and **absolute bioavailability**.

Relative availability. Relative bioavailability may be used to compare the relative absorptions of the different dosage forms of the same drug and also the relative availabilities of two different drugs with the same action when delivered using the same type of dosage form. It is defined for equal doses as:

$$\text{relative bioavailability} = \frac{\text{AUC for drug A (or dosage form A)}}{\text{AUC for drug B (or dosage form B)}} \quad (8.26)$$

Percentage relative bioavailability figures may be obtained by multiplying Equation (8.26) by 100. A correction must be made if different drug doses are used, in which case Equation (8.26) becomes:

$$\text{relative bioavailability} = \frac{(\text{AUC for drug A or dosage form A})/\text{dose A}}{(\text{AUC for drug B or dosage form B})/\text{dose B}} \quad (8.27)$$

A relative bioavailability value significantly higher than unity would suggest that the bioavailability of the drug from the dosage form A is much better than that from the dosage form B, whilst a value significantly less than unity would indicate that the reverse was true.

This type of calculation is useful in drug design as it ensures that the dosage forms used in trials are effective in delivering the drug to the general circulation. It is also used by licensing authorities as a check on the efficacy of products when manufacturers change the dosage form of a drug in clinical use.

Absolute bioavailability. Absolute bioavailability is used as a measure of the efficiency of the absorption of the drug. It is defined in terms of the total dose of the drug the body would receive if the drug were placed directly in the general circulation by an I.V. bolus injection, that is:

$$\text{absolute bioavailability}(F) = \frac{\text{AUC for oral dosage form}/\text{oral dose}}{\text{AUC for IV dosage form}/\text{IV dose}} \quad (8.28)$$

Comparison of the absolute bioavailabilities of analogues enables the medicinal chemist to select the analogue that would be most likely to give the required pharacological result. However, it should be realized that the final decision as to which analogue to develop would not be based solely on its bioavailabity. It would be based on a consideration of all the pharmacokinetic and pharmacodynamic data obtained for the three analogues.

8.5.1 Single oral dose

When a single dose of a drug is administered orally its plasma concentration increases to a maximum value (C_{max}) at t_{max} before falling with time (Figure 8.9). The increase in plasma concentration occurs as the drug is absorbed. It is accompanied by elimination, which starts from the instant the drug is absorbed. The rate of elimination increases as the concentration of the drug in the plasma increases to the maximum absorbed dose. At this point, the rate of absorption is equal to the rate of elimination. Once absorption ceases, elimination becomes the dominant pharmacokinetic factor and plasma concentration falls.

The change in plasma concentration–time curve for a single oral dose shows the time (t_{lag}) taken for the drug to reach its therapeutic window concentration, the time (t_{max}) taken to reach the maximum plasma concentration (C_{max}) and the period of time (t_{di}) for which the plasma concentration lies within the therapeutic window (Figure 8.9). However, in view of the difficulty of taking serum samples at exactly the right time both t_{max} and C_{max} are normally determined by calculation (see section 8.5.2). All these measurements are useful in determining the correct dosage form for a drug and also the selection of analogues for development.

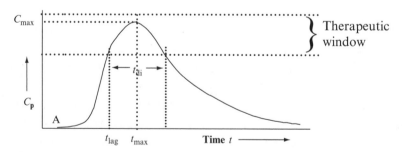

Figure 8.9   The change in plasma concentration of a drug with time due to a single oral dose of the drug. A small time lapse A occurs before the drug reaches the blood. This is mainly the time taken for the drug to reach its site of absorption from the mouth

The absorption of a drug into the general circulatory system is a complex process. Drugs given orally dissolve in the GI tract fluids before being absorbed through the GI tract membrane. The rate of absorption depends on both the drug's chemical nature and the physical conditions at the site of absorption. However, most drugs exhibit approximately first order absorption and elimination kinetics except when there is a high local concentration that saturates the absorptive and/or elimination mechanisms, in which case zero order characteristics are often found.

The rate of change of the amount (A) of an orally administered drug in the body with time will depend on the relative rates of absorption and elimination, that is:

$$dA/dt = \text{rate of absorption} - \text{rate of elimination} \qquad (8.29)$$

The changes in a drug's plasma concentration with time may be calculated for a specific pharmacokinetic model by substituting of the appropriate rate expressions into Equation (8.29). For example, for a one compartment model in which the drug exhibits first order absorption and elimination (Figure 8.10), it is possible to show that:

$$C_p = \frac{FD_0}{V_d} \frac{k_{ab}}{(k_{ab} - k_{el})} (e^{-k_{el}t} - e^{-k_{ab}t}) \qquad (8.30)$$

where k_{ab} and k_{el} are the absorption and elimination rate constants respectively and D_0 is the dose administered. The value of k_{ab} may be obtained by substituting the relevant values for F, D_0, V_d, k_{el}, and t in Equation (8.30).

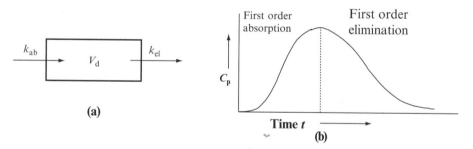

(a)

(b)

Figure 8.10   (a) A one compartment model for a single orally administered dose. (b) The plasma concentration–time curve for a drug that exhibits first order kinetics for both its absorption and elimination

Expressions similar to Equation (8.30) may be obtained for drugs that do not exhibit first order absorption and elimination characteristics by substituting the appropriate kinetic relationships in Equation (8.29). For example, for a drug that exhibits zero order absorption and first order elimination kinetics, Equation (8.29) becomes:

$$dA/dt = k_0 - k_{el}A \qquad (8.31)$$

where k_0 is the zero rate constant for the absorption process. However, it should be realised that some drug absorption and elimination processes do not exhibit zero or first order kinetics, and so these processes cannot always be so easily quantified.

8.5.2   The calculation of t_{max} and C_{max}

The calculation of t_{max} and C_{max} for a drug normally starts from the relevant equation for the change in plasma concentration of the drug with time derived from Equation (8.29). For example, for drugs that exhibit first order absorption and elimination kinetics, Equation (8.30) (see section 8.5.1) shows how C_p changes with time. Differentiation of Equation (8.30) gives:

$$\frac{dC_p}{dt} = \frac{FD_0}{V_d} \frac{k_{ab}}{(k_{ab} - k_{el})}(-k_{el}e^{-k_{el}t} + k_{ab}e^{-k_{ab}t}) \tag{8.32}$$

but at t_{max} $dC_p/dt = 0$ and so:

$$\frac{FD_0}{V_d} \frac{k_{ab}}{(k_{ab} - k_{el})}(-k_{el}e^{-k_{el}t_{max}} + k_{ab}e^{-k_{ab}t_{max}}) = 0 \tag{8.33}$$

$$\text{simplifying :} \quad -k_{el}e^{-k_{el}t_{max}} + k_{ab}e^{-k_{ab}t_{max}} = 0 \tag{8.34}$$

$$\text{and :} \quad k_{ab}e^{-k_{ab}t_{max}} = k_{el}e^{-k_{el}t_{max}} \tag{8.35}$$

$$\text{taking logs to base e :} \quad \ln k_{ab} - k_{ab}t_{max} = \ln k_{el} - k_{el}t_{max} \tag{8.36}$$

$$\text{and so :} \quad t_{max} = \frac{\ln k_{el} - \ln k_{ab}}{k_{el} - k_{ab}} \tag{8.37}$$

Once t_{max} has been calculated C_{max} can be found by substitution of the appropriate values of F, V_d, D_0, k_{ab} and k_{el} for the drug in Equation (8.30). Since F and V_d are constants C_{max} is proportional to the dose administered: the larger the dose the greater C_{max}.

8.5.3   Repeated oral doses

In order that a drug is therapeutically effective its plasma concentration must be maintained within its therapeutic window for a long enough period of time to

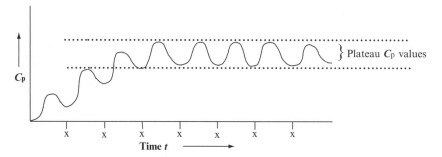

Figure 8.11 The general changes in plasma concentration with time for repeated oral doses. Repeat doses were administered at regular times intervals x

obtain the desired therapeutic effect. This can only be achieved by the use of repeat doses at regular time intervals. Initially, for each dose, the rate of absorption will exceed the rate of elimination and so the plasma concentration of the drug will steadily increase as the number of doses increases (Figure 8.11). However, as the plasma concentration increases so does the rate of elimination and so, eventually, the plasma concentration will reach a plateau. The value of the plateau plasma concentration will vary between a maximum and minimum value, the time interval between these values depending on the time interval between the doses. The values of k_{ab} and k_{el} may be used to calculate the plateau maximum and minimum drug plasma concentration values. This is useful in designing multiple dosage form regimens.

The time taken to achieve a plateau concentration may be reduced by using a larger than usual initial dose. This **loading dose**, as it is known, gives a relatively high initial plasma concentration, which acts as an elevated starting point for the succeeding normal doses. This reduces the time taken to reach the plateau concentration, that is, the therapeutic window, and so can be particularly useful in cases of serious illness.

8.6 The use of pharmacokinetics in drug design

Pharmacokinetic data is used to differentiate between active substances with good and poor pharmacokinetic characteristics. For example, substances with poor absorption, high first pass metabolism and an unsuitable half-life (too long or too short) will normally be discarded in favour of substances with more appropriate pharmacokinetic properties.

Pharmacokinetics is used in all the development stages of a drug from preclinical to Phase IV trials (see section 11.3). Legislation normally demands that the absorption, elimination, distribution, clearance, bioavailability, $t_{1/2}$ and V_d of all existing and new drugs must be defined using preclinical trials. In theory, all these parameters can be scaled up from animal experiments to predict the behaviour of the substance in humans, but the correlation is usually only approximate. The same parameters are required for Phase I trials. Phase I results for bioavailability and $t_{1/2}$ are used by the pharmaceutical industry as part of the evidence for deciding whether further investigation of a potential drug would be justified. Phase I trials are also used to predict appropriate dose levels for the expected patient community.

Once the drug has been found to be safe and effective in the Phase I trials, the evaluation of pharmacokinetic parameters is required for the diseased state, age (young and old) and gender in the Phase II trials. It is especially important to determine the effect of reduced liver and kidney function on the elimination of the new drug in order to avoid toxic effects due to the use of too high a dose level in patients with these conditions. All this information is used to develop effective safe dosage forms for new drugs and to check new dosage forms for existing drugs.

8.7 Questions

(1) Explain the meaning of each of the following terms: (a) therapeutic window; (b) IV bolus; (c) clearance and (d) first pass effect.

(2)

(A)

Megestrol acetate (A) is an oral contraceptive. What pharmacokinetic parameters should be determined for other potential oral contraceptives in order to compare their actions with compound A? Give reasons for your choice.

(3) A patient was given a single dose of 30 mg of a drug by an IV bolus injection. The drug plasma concentration was determined at set time intervals, the data obtained being recorded in Table 8.4. Calculate:

(i)   the value of the elimination constant of the drug,

(*continued*)

Table 8.4.

Time (hours)	Plasma concentration (μg cm^{-3})	Time (hours)	Plasma concentration (μg cm^{-3})
1	5.9	4	3.0
2	4.7	5	2.4
3	3.7	6	1.9

(ii) the apparent volume of distribution of the drug,
(iii) the clearance of the drug.

What fundamental assumption has to be made in order to calculate these values?

(4) The clearance of a drug from a body compartment is 5 cm^3 min^{-1}. If the compartment originally contained 50 mg of this drug, calculate the amount of drug remaining in the system after 1, 2, 3, 4, 5, 6, 7, 8, 9 and 10 minutes if the volume of the compartment was 50 cm^3. Plot a graph of concentration against time and determine the values of $t_{1/2}$ and k_{el} for the compartment and the drug.

(5) A dose of 50 mg of the drug used in question (3) was administered orally to the same patient who received the IV bolus in question (3). Plasma samples were taken at regular time intervals and a graph of plasma concentration against time plotted. If the area under this curve was 5.01, calculate the absolute bioavailability of the drug in the patient assuming first order absorption and elimination. Comment on the value of the figure obtained. You may use the IV data recorded in question (3).

(6) The data in Table 8.5 is based on plasma concentration–time curves for a number of analogues of a lead. Calculate the relevant pharmacokinetic

Table 8.5.

Analogue	Elimination rate constant minutes^{-1} (m^{-1})	AUC IV bolus (30 mg dose) μg m cm^{-3}	AUC single oral dose (30 mg dose) μg m cm^{-3}
A	0.1386	30.4	31.5
B	0.0277	31.2	47.6
C	0.0462	100.3	81.4
D	0.0173	69.7	81.9

(*continues overleaf*)

(*continued*)

parameter(s) and indicate the best analogue for further investigation if a drug with a reasonable duration of action is required. Assume that the absorption and elimination of the drug follows first order kinetics.

(7) A patient is being treated with morphine by intravenous infusion. The steady state plasma concentration of the drug is to be maintained at $0.04\,\mu g\ cm^{-3}$. Calculate the rate of infusion necessary assuming a first order elimination process (for morphine V_d is $4.0\,dm^3$ and $t_{1/2}$ is 2.5 hours).

9 Drug Metabolism

9.1 Introduction

Drug metabolism or biotransformations are the chemical reactions that are responsible for the conversion of drugs into other products (**metabolites**) within the body before and after they have reached their sites of action. It usually occurs by more than one route (Figure 9.1, R-(+)-warfarin). These routes normally consist of a series of enzyme controlled reactions. Their end products are normally pharmacologically inert compounds, which are more easily excreted than the original drug. The reactions involved in these routes are classified for convenience as **Phase I** (see section 9.4) and **Phase II** (see section 9.5) reactions. Phase I reactions either introduce or unmask functional groups, which are believed to act as a centre for Phase II reactions. The products of Phase I reactions are often more water soluble and so more readily excreted than the parent drug. Phase II reactions produce compounds that are often very water soluble and usually form the bulk of the inactive excreted products of drug metabolism.

The rate of drug metabolism controls the duration and intensity of the action of many drugs by controlling the amount of the drug reaching its target site. In addition, the metabolites produced may be pharmacologically active (see section 9.2). Consequently, it is important in the development of a new drug to document the behaviour of the metabolic products of a drug as well as that of their parent drug in the body. Furthermore, in the case of prodrugs, metabolism is also responsible for liberating the active form of the drug.

9.1.1 The stereochemistry of drug metabolism

The body contains a number of nonspecific enzymes that form part of its defence against unwanted xenobiotics. Drugs are metabolized by both these

Fundamentals of Medicinal Chemistry, Edited by Gareth Thomas
© 2003 John Wiley & Sons, Ltd
ISBN 0 470 84306 3 (Hbk), ISBN 0 470 84307 1 (pbk)

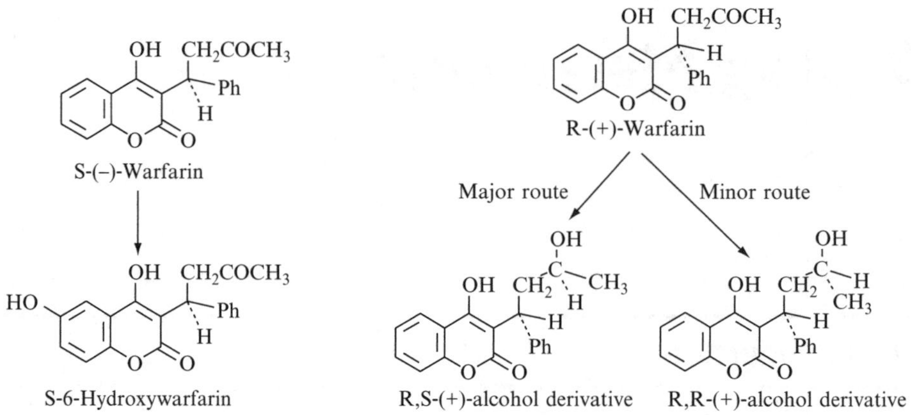

Figure 9.1   The different metabolic routes of S-(−)-warfarin and R-(+)-warfarin in humans

enzymes and the more specific enzymes that are found in the body. The latter enzymes usually catalyse the metabolism of drugs that have structures related to those of the normal substrates of the enzyme and so are to a certain extent stereospecific. The stereospecific nature of some enzymes means that enantiomers may be metabolized by different routes, in which case they could produce different metabolites (Figure 9.1).

In some cases an inert enantiomer is metabolized into its active enantiomer. For example, R-ibuprofen is inactive but is believed to be metabolized to the active analgesic S-ibuprofen.

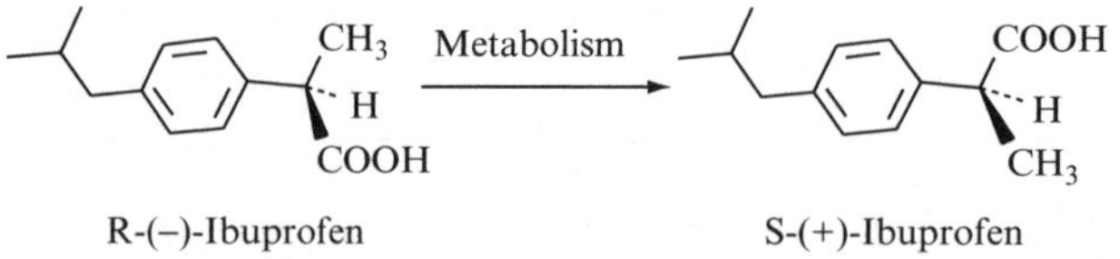

A direct consequence of the stereospecific nature of many metabolic processes is that racemic modifications must be treated as though they contained two different drugs, each with its own pharmacokinetic and pharmacodynamic properties. Investigation of these properties must include an investigation of the metabolites of each of the enantiomers of the drug. Furthermore, if a drug is going to be administered in the form of a racemic modification, the metabolism of the racemic modification must also be determined, since this could be different from that observed when the pure enantiomers are administered separately.

9.1.2 Biological factors affecting metabolism

The metabolic differences found within a species are believed to be due to variations in age, sex, genetics and diseases. In particular, diseases that affect the liver will have a large effect on drug metabolism. Diseases of organs, such as the kidneys and lungs, that are less important centres for metabolism will also affect the excretion of metabolic products. Consequently, when testing new drugs, it is essential to design trials to cover all these aspects of metabolism.

1. **Age.** The ability to metabolize drugs is lower in the very young (under 5) and the elderly (over 60). However, it is emphasized that the quoted ages are approximate and the actual changes will vary according to the individual and their lifestyle. In the foetus and the very young (neonates), many metabolic routes are not fully developed. This is because the enzymes equired by metabolic processes are not produced in sufficient quantities until several months after birth. Children (above 5) and teenagers usually have the same metabolic routes as adults. However, their smaller body volume means that smaller doses are required to achieve the desired therapeutic effect.

2. **Sex.** The metabolic pathway followed by a drug is normally the same for both males and females. However, some sex related differences in the metabolism of anxiolytics, hypnotics and a number of other drugs have been observed. Pregnant women will also exhibit changes in the rate of metabolism of some drugs. For example, the metabolism of both the analgesic pethidine and the antipsychotic chlorpromazine are reduced during pregnancy.

3. **Genetic variations.** Variations in the genetic codes of individuals can result in the absence of enzymes, low concentrations of enzymes or the formation of enzymes with reduced activity. These differences in enzyme concentration and activity result in individuals exhibiting different metabolic rates and in some cases different pharmacological responses for the same drug. An individual's inability to metabolize a drug could result in that drug accumulating in the body. This could give rise to unwanted effects.

9.1.3 Environmental factors affecting metabolism

The metabolism of a drug is also affected by lifestyle. Poor diet, drinking, smoking and drug abuse may all have an influence on the rate of metabolism. The use of over-the-counter self-medicaments may also affect the rate of metabolism of an endogenous ligand or a prescribed drug. Since the use of over-the-counter medicaments is widespread, it can be difficult to assess the results of some large scale clinical trials.

9.1.4 Species and metabolism

Different species often respond differently to a drug. This is believed to be due to differences in metabolism between species. These metabolic differences may take the form of either different metabolic pathways for the same compound or different rates of metabolism when the pathway is the same. Both deviations are though to be largely due to enzyme deficiencies or sufficiencies.

9.2 Secondary pharmacological implications of metabolism

Metabolites may be either pharmacologically inactive or active. Active metabolites may exhibit a similar activity to the drug or a different activity or be toxic (Table 9.1). In addition, they may exhibit different side effects.

9.3 Sites of action

Drug metabolism can occur in all tissues and most biological fluids. However, the widest range of metabolic reactions occurs in the liver. A more substrate-selective range of metabolic processes takes place in the kidney, lungs, brain, placenta and other tissues.

Orally administered drugs may be metabolized as soon as they are ingested. However, the first region where a significant degree of drug metabolism occurs is usually in the GI tract and within the intestinal wall. Once absorbed from the GI tract, many potential and existing drugs are extensively metabolized by first pass metabolism (see section 8.5). For example, the first pass metabolism of

Table 9.1 Some of the types of secondary pharmaceutical activity of metabolites. Note that not all the possible metabolic routes for a drug are given in the examples

Metabolite activity	Example and notes
Inactive	Routes that result in the formation of inactive metabolites are often referred to as detoxification
Similar activity to the drug	The metabolite may exhibit either a different potency or duration of action or both to the original drug.
Different activity	
Toxic metabolites	

some drugs such as lignocaine is so complete that they cannot be administered orally. The bioavailability of other drugs, such as nitroglycerine (vasodilator), propranolol (antihypertensive) and pethidine (narcotic analgesic), is significantly reduced by their first pass metabolism.

9.4   Phase I metabolic reactions

The main Phase I reactions are biological oxidations, reductions, hydrolyses, hydrations, deacetylations and isomerizations, although a wide range of other reactions are included in this category. A knowledge of these biological reactions and the structure of a molecule makes it possible to predict its most likely metabolic products. However, the complex nature of biological systems makes an accurate comprehensive prediction difficult. As a result, the identification of the metabolites of a drug and their significance is normally determined by experiment during its preclinical and Phase I trials. Prediction of the possible products can be of some help in these identifications, although it should not be allowed to obscure the possible existence of unpredicted metabolites. Furthermore, computer based prediction systems are becoming available but lack sufficient data to fully predict the metabolic route of a specific compound from its structure.

9.4.1   Oxidation

Oxidation is by far the most important Phase I metabolic reaction. One of the main enzyme systems involved in the oxidation of xenobiotics appears to be the so called **mixed function oxidases** or **monooxygenases**, which are found mainly in the smooth endoplasmic reticulum of the liver but also occur, to a lesser extent, in other tissues. These enzymes tend to be nonspecific, catalysing the metabolism of a wide variety of compounds (Table 9.2). Two common mixed function oxidase systems are the cytochrome P-450 (CYP-450) and the flavin monooxygenase (FMO) systems (Appendix 12). The overall oxidations of these systems take place in a series of oxidative and reductive steps, each step being catalysed by a specific enzyme. Many of these steps require the presence of molecular oxygen and either NADH or NADPH as co-enzymes.

A number of other enzymes, such as monoamine oxidase, alcohol dehydrogenase and xanthine oxidase, are also involved in drug metabolism. These enzymes tend to be more specific, oxidizing xenobiotics related to the normal substrate for the enzyme.

9.4.2   Reduction

Reduction is an important reaction for the metabolism of compounds that contain reducible groups, such as aldehydes, ketones, alkenes, nitro groups,

Table 9.2 Examples of mixed function oxidase catalysed oxidations. Oxidation introduces or reveals new functional groups (shaded). Note: these reactions are not the only routes for the metabolism of the drugs used as examples

Type of reaction (groups)	Example
Aromatic hydroxylation (aromatic C–H)	Lignocaine (local anaesthetic)
Aliphatic hydroxylation (aliphatic C–H)	Pentobarbitone (sedative, hypnotic)
Epoxidization (aromatic and alkene groups)	Carbamazepine (anticonvulsant)

(continues overleaf)

Table 9.2   *(continued)*

Type of reaction (groups)	Example

Dealkylation
(methyl and ethyl secondary amines, tertiary amines, ethers and thioethers. The methanal and ethanal produced are often excreted via the lungs, giving the patient bad breath.)

Imipramine (antidepressant) $(CH_2)_3N(CH_3)_2$
$\xrightarrow{HCHO}$
Desmethylimipramine (antipsychotic) $(CH_2)_3$ NH CH_3
$\xrightarrow{HCHO}$
$(CH_2)_3$ NH₂

Phenacetin (analgesic) CH_3CH_2O —NHCOCH₃
$\xrightarrow{CH_3CHO}$
Paracetamol (analgesic) HO —NHCOCH₃

6–Methylthiopurine SCH₃
$\xrightarrow{}$
6–Mercaptopurine (anticancer) SH + HCHO

Oxidative dehalogenation
The reactive electrophilic acyl and carbonyl compounds produced by oxidative dehalogenation may react with nucleophilic biological molecules such as DNA, proteins, lipids and carbohydrates to possibly form toxic metabolites.

Chloramphenicol (antibiotic) O_2N— CH–CH— NH–C–C–C–Cl
$\xrightarrow{}$
O_2N— CH–CH— NH–C–C + HCl

Highly reactive xamyl chloride derivative

azo groups and sulphoxides. The enzymes used to catalyse metabolic reductions are usually specific in their action. Many of them require NADPH as a coenzyme. Reduction of some functional groups results in the formation of stereoisomers. Although this means that two metabolic routes may be necessary to deal with the products of the reduction, only one product usually predominates. For example, R(+)-warfarin is reduced to a mixture of the corresponding RS(+) and RR(+) diastereoisomers, the RS(+) isomer being the major product.

R(+)–Warfarin   1R,3S(+)–Alcohol (major product)   1R,3S(+)–Alcohol (minor product)

9.4.3 Hydrolysis

Hydrolysis is an important metabolic reaction for drugs whose structures contain ester and amide groups. All types of ester and amide can be metabolized by this route. Ester hydrolysis is often catalysed by specific esterases in the liver, kidney and other tissues as well as non-specific esterases such as acetylcholinesterases and pseudocholinesterases in the plasma. Amide hydrolysis is also catalysed by non-specific esterases in the plasma as well as amidases in the liver. More specific enzyme systems are able to hydrolyse sulphate and glucuronate conjugates as well as hydrate epoxides, glycosides and other moieties.

The hydrolysis of esters is usually rapid whilst that of amides if often much slower. This makes esters suitable as prodrugs (see Section 9.8) and amides a potential source for slow release drugs.

9.4.4 Hydration

Hydration, in the context of metabolism, is the addition of water to a structure. Epoxides are readily hydrated to diols (see carbamazepine, Table 9.1), the reaction being catalysed by the enzyme epoxide hydrolase.

9.4.5 Other Phase I reactions

The reactions involved in Phase I metabolism are not limited to those discussed in the previous sections. In theory, any suitable organic reaction could be

utilized in a metabolic route. For example, the initial stage in the metabolism of
L-dopa is decarboxylation.

9.5   Phase II metabolic routes

Phase II reactions, which are also known as **conjugation reactions**, may occur at
any point in the metabolism of a drug or xenobiotic. However, they often
represent the final step in the metabolic pathway before excretion. The products
of Phase II reactions, which are referred to as **conjugates**, are usually pharmacologically inactive, although there are some notable exceptions. They are
usually excreted in the urine and/or bile.

The reactions commonly involved in Phase II conjugation are acylation,
sulphate formation and conjugation with amino acids, glucuronic acid, glutathione and mercapturic acid (Table 9.3). Methylation is also regarded as a
Phase II reaction although it is normally a minor metabolic route. However, it
can be a major route for phenolic hydroxy groups. In all cases, the reaction is
usually catalysed by a specific transferase.

9.6   Pharmacokinetics of metabolites

The activity and behaviour of a metabolite will have a direct bearing on the safe
use and dose of a drug administered to a patient. Consequently, when investigating the pharmacokinetics of a drug it is also necessary to obtain pharmacokinetic data concerning the action and elimination of its metabolites. This
information is usually obtained in humans by administering the drug and
measuring the change in concentration of the appropriate metabolite with
time in the plasma. However, as metabolites are produced in the appropriate
body compartment, a metabolite may be partly or fully metabolized before it
reaches the plasma. In these cases the amount of metabolite found by analysis of
plasma samples is only a fraction of the amount of the metabolite produced
by the body. For simplicity, the discussions in this text assume that **all** the

Table 9.3 Phase II reactions. These normally produce pharmacologically inert metabolites but a few metabolites, such as N-acetylisoniazid and the sulphate conjugates of phenacetin, are toxic

Phase II reaction. Functional group/notes	General reaction	Example

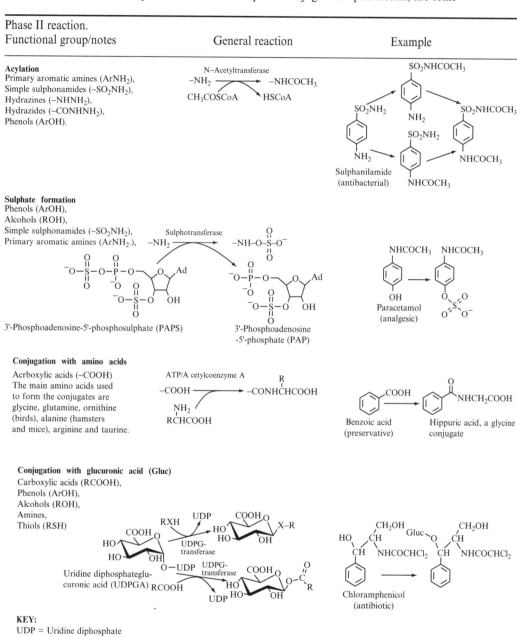

Acylation
Primary aromatic amines (ArNH₂),
Simple sulphonamides (–SO₂NH₂),
Hydrazines (–NHNH₂),
Hydrazides (–CONHNH₂),
Phenols (ArOH).

Sulphate formation
Phenols (ArOH),
Alcohols (ROH),
Simple sulphonamides (–SO₂NH₂.),
Primary aromatic amines (ArNH₂.),

3'-Phosphoadenosine-5'-phosphosulphate (PAPS)

Conjugation with amino acids

Acrboxylic acids (–COOH)
The main amino acids used
to form the conjugates are
glycine, glutamine, ornithine
(birds), alanine (hamsters
and mice), arginine and taurine.

Conjugation with glucuronic acid (Gluc)
Carboxylic acids (RCOOH),
Phenols (ArOH),
Alcohols (ROH),
Amines,
Thiols (RSH)

Uridine diphosphateglu-
curonic acid (UDPGA)

KEY:
UDP = Uridine diphosphate

(continues overleaf)

Table 9.3 (*continued*)

Phase II reaction. Functional group/notes	General reaction	Example
Conjugation with glutathione (GSH) Electrophilic centres caused by Halides, Nitro groups, Epoxides, Sulphonates, Organophosphate groups.	Electrophile $\xrightarrow[\text{GSH}]{\text{Glutathione S-transferase}}$ Electrophile-SG	Ethacrynic acid (diuretic)
Methylation Phenols (ArOH), Alcohols (ROH), Amines, N-heterocyclics. Methylation detoxifies a drug but produces a less polar and so less easily excreted metabolite.	S-adenosylmethionine (SAM) RXH $\xrightarrow{\text{X-Methyltransferase}}$ RXCH$_3$ Dimercaprol (Heavy metal poisoning antidote)	$\xrightarrow[\text{S-Methyltransferase}]{\text{SAM}}$

metabolite produced reaches the plasma. Alternatively, the metabolite may be administered separately when independent data concerning its activity and pharmacokinetics is required. However, observations made from metabolite administration can be suspect because its bioavailability is usually different to that when it is produced *in situ* from the drug.

The total administered dose (A) of a drug is excreted partly unchanged and partly metabolized (Figure 9.2). Most metabolic pathways consist of a series of steps. The importance of this series is not the number of steps but whether the pathway has a rate determining step. In other words, is there a metabolite bottleneck where the rate of elimination of a metabolite is far slower than its rate of formation from the drug? At such a point the concentration of the metabolite would increase to significant amounts, which could lead to potential clinical problems if the metabolite were pharmaceutically active. Consequently, to avoid problems of this nature a metabolite should be eliminated faster than

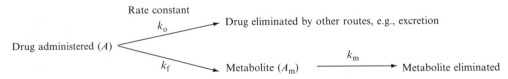

Figure 9.2 A schematic representation of the possible elimination routes for a drug in the body

the drug. The rate of change of concentration of a metabolite (dM/dt) in the plasma is given by:

$$dM/dt = \text{rate of formation} - \text{rate of elimination} \qquad (9.1)$$

Since most biological processes exhibit first order kinetics Equation (9.1) becomes:

$$dM/dt = k_f A - k_m A_m \qquad (9.2)$$

where k_f and k_m are the rate constants for the metabolite's formation and elimination processes respectively. If $k_f > k_m$ there will be an accumulation of the metabolite in the patient. However, it is not easy to determine k_f. Therefore, as all the processes involved in drug elimination are normally first order, the k overall rate constant for all the processes is used because $k = k_f + k_0$ and it is relatively easy to determine. Consequently, if $k > k_m$ the metabolite will be **likely** to accumulate in the plasma as it is formed faster than it is eliminated. However, if $k < k_m$ the metabolite is **unlikely** to accumulate in the body as the metabolite is eliminated faster than it is formed. The values of k and k_m can be determined experimentally from log plots of plasma measurements of the drug and metabolite (Figure 9.3).

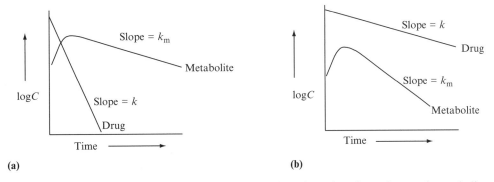

(a)   (b)

Figure 9.3 Representations of typical log concentration–time plots for a drug and metabolite exhibiting first order kinetics showing the general changes when (a) $k > k_m$ and (b) $k < k_m$

9.7 Drug metabolism and drug design

A knowledge of the metabolic pathway of a drug may be used to design analogues that have a different metabolism to that of the lead. This change of metabolism is achieved by modifying the structure of the drug. These structural modifications may either make the analogue more stable or increase its ease of metabolism relative to the lead (see Table 9.4). The structural modifications should be selected so that they do not change the nature of the pharmacological activity of the drug. However, it is not possible to accurately predict whether this will be the case and so normally the activity of the analogue may only be found by experiment.

Changing the metabolism of a lead may result in an analogue which exhibits a different type of activity to that of the lead. For example, the replacement of the ester group in the local anaesthetic procaine by an amide group produced procainamide, which acts as an antiarrhythmic (Figure 9.4(a)). It may also be used to develop analogues that do not have undesireable side effects. For example, the local anaesthetic lignocaine is also used as an antiarrhythmic. In this respect, its undesirable convulsant and emetic side effects are caused by its metabolism in the liver by dealkylation to the mono-N-ethyl derivative (Figure 9.4(b)). The removal of the N-ethyl substituents and their replacement by an α-methyl group gives the antiarrhythmic tocainide. Tocainide cannot be metabolized by the same pathway as lignocaine and does not exhibit convulsant and emetic side effects.

Table 9.4 Examples of the effect of structural modifications on the metabolism of a lead compound

Change	Structural modification
Increased metabolic stability	Replace a reactive group by a less reactive group. For example, N-dealkylation can be prevented by replacing a N-methyl group by a N-t-butyl group. Reactive ester groups are replaced by less reactive amide groups. Oxidation of aromatic rings may be reduced by introducing strong electron acceptor substituents such as chloro ($-Cl$), quaternary amine ($-\overset{+}{N}R_3$), carboxylic acid ($-COOH$), sulphonate ($-SO_3R$) and sulphonamide ($-SO_2NHR$) groups.
Decreasing metabolic stability	The ease of metabolism of a drug may be increased by incorporating a metabolically labile group, such as an ester, in the structure of the drug. This type of approach is the basis of prodrug design (see section 9.8). It has also led to the development of so called *soft drugs*. These are biologically active compounds that are rapidly metabolized by a predictable route to pharmacologically nontoxic compounds. The advantage of this type of drug is that its half-life is so short that the possibility of the patient receiving a fatal overdose is considerably reduced.

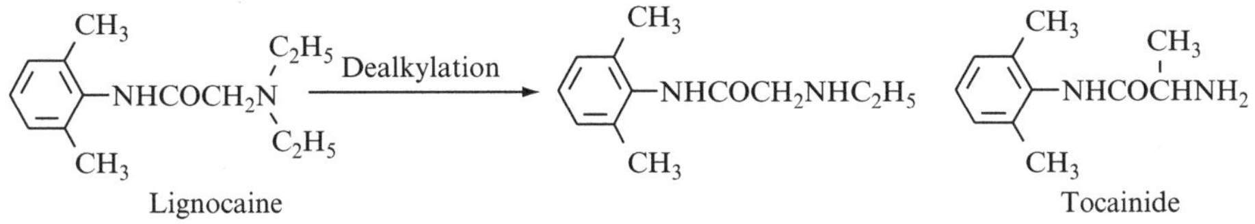

Figure 9.4 Examples of structural modifications causing changes in activity

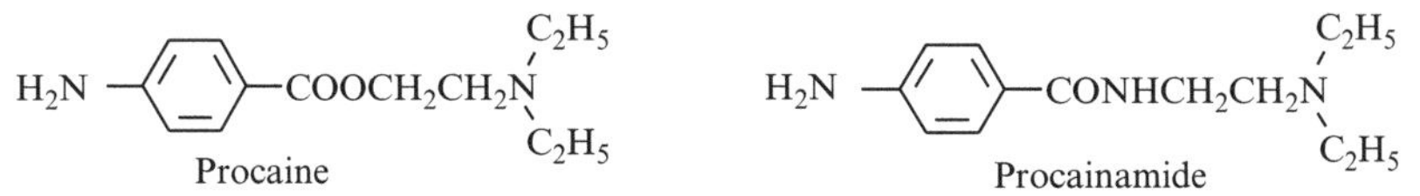

9.8 Prodrugs

Prodrugs are compounds that are biologically inactive but are metabolized to an active metabolite, which is responsible for the drug's action. They are classified as either **bioprecursor** or **carrier prodrugs**. Prodrugs may be designed to improve absorption, improve patient acceptance, reduce toxicity and also for the slow release of drugs in the body. A number of prodrugs have also been designed to be site specific (see section 9.8.3).

9.8.1 Bioprecursor prodrugs

Bioprecursor prodrugs are compounds that already contain the embryo of the active species within their structure. This active species is liberated by metabolism of the prodrug (Figure 9.5).

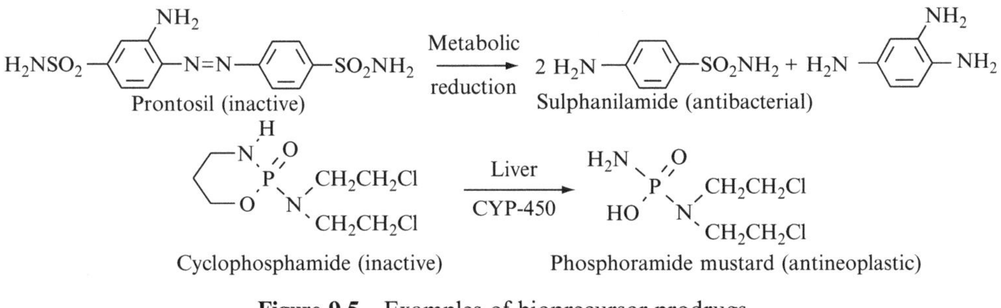

Figure 9.5 Examples of bioprecursor prodrugs

9.8.2 Carrier prodrugs

Carrier prodrugs are formed by combining an active drug with a carrier species to form a compound with the desired chemical and biological characteristics, for example, a lipophilic moiety to improve transport through membranes. The link between carrier and active species must be a group, such as an ester or amide, that can be easily metabolized once absorption has occurred or the drug has been delivered to the required body compartment. The overall process may be summarized by:

$$\text{Carrier + Active species} \xrightarrow{\quad\text{Synthesis}\quad} \text{Carrier prodrug} \xrightleftharpoons{\quad\text{Metabolism}\quad} \text{Carrier + Active species}$$

Carrier prodrugs that consist of the drug linked by a functional group to the carrier are known as **bipartate prodrugs** (Figure 9.6). **Tripartate prodrugs** are those in which the carrier is linked to the drug by a link consisting of a separate structure. In these systems, the carrier is removed by an enzyme controlled metabolic process and the linking structure by either an enzyme system or a chemical reaction.

The choice of functional group used as a metabolic link depends both on the functional groups occurring in the drug molecule (Table 9.5) and the need for the prodrug to be metabolized in the appropriate body compartment.

The precise nature of the structure of the carrier used to form a carrier prodrug will depend on the intended outcome (see section 9.8.3).

Table 9.5 Examples of the functional groups used to link carriers with drugs

Drug group (D–X)	Type of group linking carrier to the drug	Examples of R groups
Alcohol, phenol (D–OH)	Ester: D–OCOR	Alkyl, Phenyl, $-(CH_2)_2NR_2$, $-(CH_2)_n$ CONR'R'', $-(CH_2)_n$NHCOR, $-CH_2$OCOR'.
Amines (all types), imides and amides (>NH)	Amide: >NCOR	Alkyl, Phenyl, $-CH_2$NHCOAr, $-CH_2$OCOR''.
	Carbamate: >NCOR	$-OCHR'OCOR''$, $-OCH_2OPO_2H_3$.
	Imine: $>N = CHR$	Aryl.
Aldehydes and ketones ($>C = O$)	Acetals: $>C(OR)_2$	Alkyl,
	Imine: $>C = NR$	Aryl, $-$ OR.
Carboxylic acids (D–COOH)	Ester: D–COOR	Alkyl, Aryl, $-(CH_2)_n$NR'R'', $-(CH_2)_n$CONR'R'', $-(CH_2)_n$NHCOR'R'', $-$ CH(R)OCOR, $-$ CH(R)OCONR'R''.

9.8.3 The design of prodrug systems for specific purposes

The introduction of a carrier into the structure of a drug to form a prodrug may be used to change a drug's bioavailability. In some cases has been used to direct the drug to specific areas.

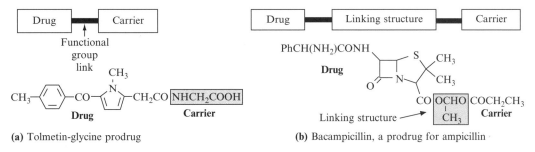

(a) Tolmetin-glycine prodrug

(b) Bacampicillin, a prodrug for ampicillin

Figure 9.6   Examples of (a) bipartate and (b) tripartate prodrug systems

Improving absorption and transport through membranes

The transport of a drug through a membrane depends largely on its relative solubilities in water and lipids (see section 2.7.1). Good absorption requires that a drug's hydrophilic–lipophilic nature is in balance. The lipophilic nature of a drug may be improved by combining a lipophilic carrier with a polar group(s) on the drug (Table 9.6). However, it is difficult to select a lipophilic carrier that will provide the degree of lipophilic character required. If the carrier is too lipophilic, the prodrug will tend to remain in the membrane. Similarly, improving the water solubility of a drug may be carried out by introducing a carrier with a water solubilizing group or groups.

Table 9.6   Examples of the reactions used to improve the lipophilic nature of drugs

Functional group	Derivative
Acids	an appropriate ester
Alcohols and phenols	an appropriate ester
Aldehydes	acetal
Ketones	acetal (ketal)
Amines	quaternary ammonium derivatives, amino acid peptides and imines

Improving patient acceptance

Odour and taste are important aspects of drug administration. A drug with a poor odour or too bitter a taste will be rejected by patients, especially children. Furthermore, a drug that causes pain when administered by injection can have a detrimental effect on a patient. The formation of a carrier prodrug can sometimes alleviate some of these problems. For example, palmitic acid and other long chain fatty acids are often used as carriers, since they usually form prodrugs with a bland taste.

Slow release

Prodrugs may be used to prolong the duration of action by providing a slow release mechanism for the drug. Slow release and subsequent extension of action is often provided by the slow hydrolysis of amide and ester linked fatty acid carriers. Hydrolysis of these groups can release the drug over a period of time that can vary from several hours to weeks. For example, the use of glycine as a carrier for the anti-inflammatory tolmetin sodium results in the duration of its peak concentration being increased from about one to nine hours.

Tolmetin sodium   Tolmetin-glycine prodrug

Site specificity

In theory, it should be possible to design a carrier prodrug that would only release the drug in the vicinity of its site of action. Furthermore, once released, the drug should remain mainly in the target area and only slowly migrate to other areas. In addition the carrier should be metabolized to nontoxic metabolites. Unfortunately, these requirements have only been achieved in a few cases.

One area where the site specific carrier prodrug approach has been used with some degree of success is to design drugs capable of crossing the blood–brain barrier (Appendix 11). This barrier will only allow the passage of very lipophilic molecules unless there is an active transport mechanism available for the compound. A method developed by Bodor and other workers involved the combination of a hydrophilic drug with a suitable lipophilic carrier, which after crossing the blood–brain barrier would be rapidly metabolized to the drug and carrier. Once released, the hydrophilic drug is unable to recross the blood–brain barrier. The selected carrier must also be metabolized to yield nontoxic metabolites. Carriers based on the dihydropyridine ring system have been found to be particularly useful in this respect. This ring system has been found to have the required lipophilic character for crossing not only the blood–brain barrier but also other membrane barriers. The dihydropyridine system is particularly useful, since it is possible to vary the functional groups attached to the dihydropyridine ring, so that the carrier can be designed to link to a specific drug. Once the dihydropyridine prodrug has crossed the blood–brain barrier it is easily oxidized by the oxidases found in the brain to the hydrophilic quaternary ammonium salt, which cannot return across the barrier, and relatively nontoxic pyridine derivatives in the vicinity of its site of action.

A method of approach followed by some workers is to design prodrugs that are activated by enzymes that are found mainly at the target site. This strategy has been used to design antitumour drugs, since tumours contain higher proportions of phosphatases and peptidases than normal tissues. For example, diethylstilbestrol diphosphate (Fosfestrol) has been used to deliver the oestrogen agonist diethylstilbestrol to prostatic carcinomas.

Unfortunately this approach has not been very successful for producing site specific antitumour drugs. However, site specific prodrugs have been developed to deliver drugs to a number of sites.

9.8.3.5 Minimizing side effects

Prodrug formation may be used to minimize toxic side effects. For example, salicylic acid is one of the oldest analgesics known. However, its use can cause gastric irritation and bleeding. The conversion of salicylic acid to its prodrug aspirin by acetylation of the phenolic hydroxy group of salicylic acid improves absorption and also reduces the degree of stomach irritation, since aspirin is mainly converted to salicylic acid by esterases after absorption from the GI tract. This reduces the amount of salicylic acid in contact with the gut wall lining.

Salicylic acid   Aspirin

9.9 Questions

(1) Explain the significance of each of the members of following pairs of terms: (a) Phase I and Phase II reactions and (b) carrier and bioprecursor prodrugs.

(2) List the main biological factors that could influence drug metabolism. Outline their main effects.

(3) Outline the types of pharmacological activity that a metabolite could exhibit.

(4) Outline, by means of general equations, how conjugation with glycine is used to metabolize aromatic acids. Suggest a chemical reason for the product of this process being readily excreted by the kidney.

(5) Suggest, by means of chemical equations and/or notes, feasible initial steps for the metabolism of each of the following compounds: (a) pethidine and (b) 4-aminoazobenzene.

(6) (a) What is the desired objective of drug metabolism? How is this normally achieved?

   (b) Suggest a series of metabolic reactions that could form a feasible metabolic pathway for N,N-dimethyl aminobenzene.

(*continued*)

(7) The following scheme represents the hypothetical metabolic pathway of a drug. The figures in brackets are the rate constants for the appropriate step.

$$\text{Drug} \xrightarrow{(0.04)} \text{A} \xrightarrow{(0.30)} \text{B} \xrightarrow{(4.67)} \text{C} \xrightarrow{(0.004)} \text{D} \xrightarrow{(2.49)} \text{E} \longrightarrow \text{Excreted}$$

$$\text{B} \xrightarrow{(0.04)} \text{F} \longrightarrow \text{Excreted}$$

(a) Explain the significance of the rate constants for the metabolism of the drug to stage B.

(b) What is the significance of the rate constants for the metabolism of B to F and C respectively?

(c) Where is the rate determining step of the series? What is its significance?

(8) Why is it necessary to design drugs with a very rapid rate of metabolism?

(9) Design a prodrug that could be used to transport the diethanoate ester of dopamine (A) across the blood–brain barrier. Show by means of notes and equations how this prodrug would function.

10 An Introduction to Lead and Analogue Syntheses

10.1 Introduction

Once the structure of a lead has been decided it is necessary to design a synthetic pathway to produce that lead. These pathways may be broadly classified as either **partial** or **full** synthetic routes. However, partial synthetic routes tend to be more concerned with the large scale production of proven drugs rather than the synthesis of lead compounds. This chapter is intended to introduce some of the strategies used, and the challenges associated with the design of these synthetic routes.

Partial synthetic pathways use biochemical and other methods to produce the initial starting materials and traditional organic synthesis to convert these compounds to the target structure. These methods are used to produce the initial starting materials because it usually cuts down the cost of production and produces compounds whose structures have the required configurations. For example, the total synthesis of steroidal drugs is not feasible because of the many chiral centres found in their structures. Consequently, partial synthesis is the normal approach to producing new analogues and manufacturing steroidal drugs. For example, the starting material for the production of progesterone is diosgenin obtained from a number of *Dioscorea species* (a plant source). Diosgenin may beconverted to pregnenolone ethanoate by a series of steps (Figure 10.1). This compound serves as the starting material for the synthesis of a number of steroidal drugs including progesterone.

The full synthetic routes start with readily available compounds, both synthetic and naturally occurring, but only utilize the standard methods of organic synthesis to produce the desired product. These methods are discussed in sections 10.2 and 10.3.

Fundamentals of Medicinal Chemistry, Edited by Gareth Thomas
© 2003 John Wiley & Sons, Ltd
ISBN 0 470 84306 3 (Hbk), ISBN 0 470 84307 1 (pbk)

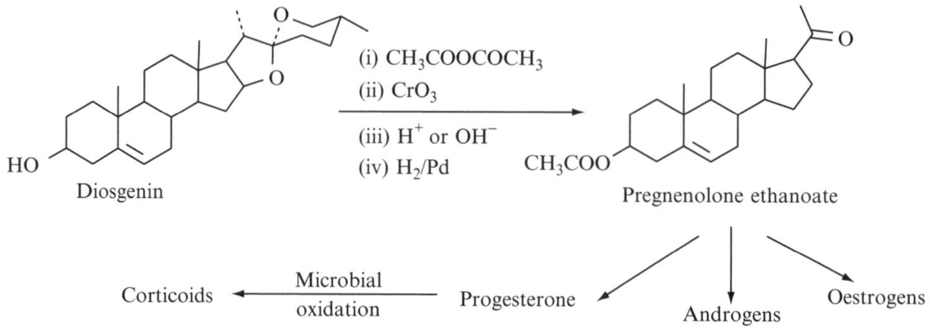

Figure 10.1   An outline of the synthesis of progesterone from diosgenin

All approaches are based on a knowledge of the chemistry of functional groups and their associated carbon skeletons. The design may be either a **linear synthesis**, where one step in the pathway is immediately followed by another, or a **convergent synthesis**, where two or more sections of the molecule are synthesized separately before being combined to form the target structure (Figure 10.2). Each of these approaches may involve steps where protecting groups have to be used. These groups should be selected on the basis that they are easy to attach, stable under the conditions that are used for the primary reaction and easy to remove after the primary reaction(s) have been completed.

In both linear and convergent synthesis designs, common sense dictates that the starting materials should be chosen on the basis of what will give the best chance of reaching the desired product. In addition, they should be cheap and

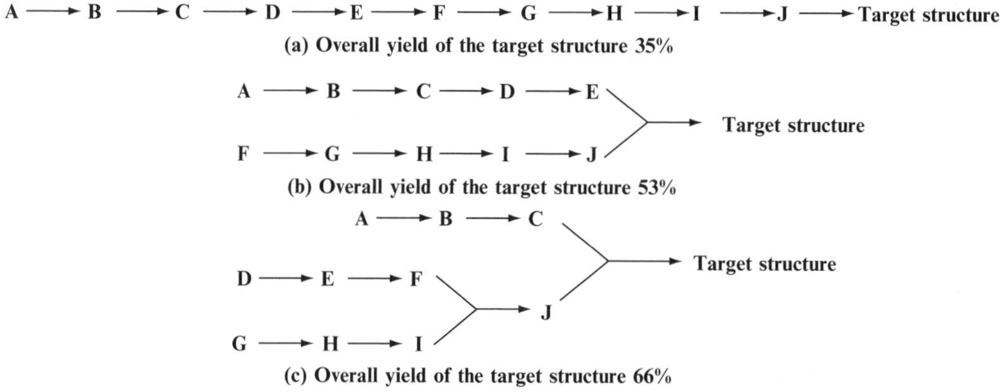

Figure 10.2   A schematic representation of (a) linear and (b) and (c) convergent syntheses. The overall yields are based on a 90% yield for each step. In general, convergent synthesis improves the overall yield of the target structure

readily available. The **disconnection** approach (see section 10.3.1) may be used both to identify these starting materials and to define the steps in the pathway. Alternatively, suitable starting compounds and a route may be determined by modification of the known synthetic route for a compound with a similar structure to the target.

The chemical reactions selected for the proposed synthetic pathway will obviously depend on the structure of the target compound. However, a number of general considerations need to be borne in mind when selecting these reactions.

1. The yields of reactions should be high. This is particularly important when the synthetic pathway involves a large number of steps.

2. The products should be relatively easy to isolate purify and identify.

3. Reactions should be stereospecific, as it is often difficult and expensive to separate enantiomers. This is a condition that is often difficult to satisfy.

4. The reactions used in the research stage of the synthesis should be adaptable to large scale production methods (see section 11.2).

An important aspect of all medicinal chemistry synthetic pathway design is divergency. Ideally, the chosen route should be such that it is relatively easy to modify the structure of the lead compound either directly or during the course of its synthesis. This is an economic way of producing a greater range of analogues for testing and hence increasing the chance of discovering anactive compound. Initially these modifications would normally take the form of changing the nature of side chains or introducing new substituents in previously unsubstituted positions. The synthetic pathway for the preparation of the lead compound should include stages where it is possible to introduce these new side chains and substituents. For example, the presence of an amino group in a structure opens out the possibility of introducing different side chains by N-acylation (Figure 10.3).

10.2   Asymmetry in syntheses

The presence of a asymmetric centre or centres in a target structure means that its synthesis requires either the use of **non-stereoselective reactions** and the

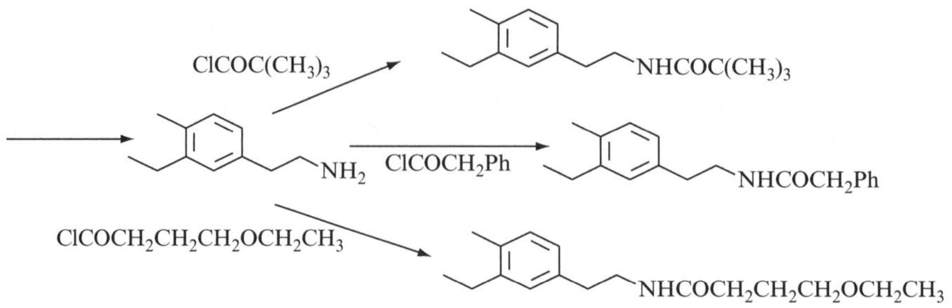

Figure 10.3 A stage in a hypothetical drug design pathway illustrating some of the possibilities provided by the presence of an amino group in the structure of an intermediate. The products of the reactions illustrated could be either the final products of the design pathway or they could be intermediates for the next stage(s) in the synthetic pathway

separation of the resulting stereoisomers or the use of **stereoselective reactions** that mainly produce one of the possible enantiomers. This section introduces some of the general methods used to incorporate stereospecific centres into a target molecule. However, for a more comprehensive discussion the reader is referred to *Selectivity in Organic Synthesis* by R. S. Ward, published by Wiley (1999).

10.2.1 The use of non-stereoselective reactions to produce stereospecific centres

Non-stereoselective reactions produce either a mixture of diastereoisomers or a racemic modification. Diastereoisomers exhibit different physical properties. Consequently, techniques utilizing these differences may be used to separate the isomers. The most common methods of separation are fractional crystallization and chromatography.

The separation (**resolution**) of a racemic modification into its constituent enantiomers is normally achieved by converting the enantiomers in the racemate into a pair of diastereoisomers by reaction with a pure enantiomer (Figure 10.4.). Enantiomers of acids are used for racemates of bases whilst enantiomers of bases are used for racemates of acids (Table 10.1). Neutral compounds may sometimes be resolved by conversion to an acidic or basic derivative which is suitable for diastereoisomer formation. The diastereoisomers are separated using methods based on the differences in their physical properties and the pure enantiomers are regenerated from the corresponding diastereoisomers by suitable reactions.

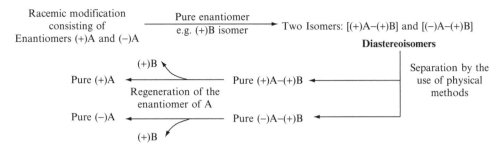

Figure 10.4 A Schematic representation of the use of diastereoisomers in the resolution of racemic modifications

Table 10.1 Examples of the pure enantiomers used to resolve racemic modifications by forming diastereoisomers. In all regeneration processes there is a danger of the racemic modification being reformed by racemization

Functional group	Enantiomers used (resolving agents)	Diastereoisomers	Regeneration
Carboxylic and other acids	A suitable base, e.g.	Salts	Treatment with a suitable acid, e.g. HCl
	(−) Brucine		
	(−) Strychnine		
	(−) Morphine		
Amines and other bases	A suitable acid, e.g.	Salts	Treatment with a suitable base, e.g. NaOH
	(+) Tartaric acid		
	(−) Malic acid		
	(+) Camphorsulphonic acid		
Alcohols	A suitable acid (see above)	Esters	Acid or base hydrolysis

The incorporation of the resolution of a racemic modification into a synthetic pathway considerably reduces the overall yield of the synthesis because the maximum theoretical yield of an enantiomer is 50 per cent unless the unwanted enantiomer is racemized and the racemate recycled.

10. 2. 2   The use of stereoselective reactions to produce stereospecific centres

Stereoselective reactions are those that result in the selective production of one of the stereoisomers of the product. The extent of the selectivity may be recorded as the **enantiomeric excess** (e.e.) when the reaction produces a mixture of enantiomers and the **diastereoisomeric excess** (d.e.) when it produces a mixture of diastereoisomers. These quantities are defined by the expression:

$$\text{e.e. or d.e.} = \frac{(\text{yield of the major stereoisomer} - \text{yield of the minor stereoisomer})}{\text{yield of the major stereoisomer} + \text{yield of the minor stereoisomer}} \times 100 \quad (10.1)$$

that is:

$$\text{e.e. or d.e.} = \%\,\text{major stereoisomer} - \%\,\text{minor isomer} \quad (10.2)$$

The values of e.e. and d.e. are obtained by measuring the yields of the individual stereoisomers. An e.e. or d.e. value of 0 per cent means that the stereoisomers are produced in equal amounts. In the case of enantiomeric mixtures the product is likely to be in the form of a racemic modification. Conversely, an e.e. or d.e. value of 100% indicates that only one product is formed. This rarely occurs in practice since most reactions yield a mixture of isomers.

The stereochemistry of the product of a reaction will be influenced by the structures of the reagent and substrate and the mechanisms by which they react. For example, the hydroxylation of but-2-ene by osmium tetroxide and water yields a racemate whilst bromination of the same compound with bromine produces a meso compound (Figure 10.5). However, a stereoselective reaction is most likely to occur when steric hindrance at the reaction centre restricts the approach of the reagent to one direction (Figure 10.6). Furthermore, the action of both enzyme and non-enzyme catalysts may also be used to introduce specific stereochemical centres into a molecule.

In reactions that produce diastereoisomers the relative proportions of the diastereoisomers produced will depend on the relative values of the activation energies of the pathways producing the stereoisomers. The greater the difference in these activation energies, the higher the possibility of the reaction being diastereoselective with respect to the product formed by the lowest activation energy pathway. Consequently, lowering the reaction temperature will often favour the formation of the diastereoisomer with the lowest activation energy.

10.2.3 General methods of asymmetric synthesis

There is no set method for designing an asymmetric synthesis. Each synthesis must be treated on its merits and in all cases success will depend on the skill and ingenuity of the research worker.

The range and scope of the reactions used in asymmetric synthesis is extremely large and consequently difficult to classify. In this text they are

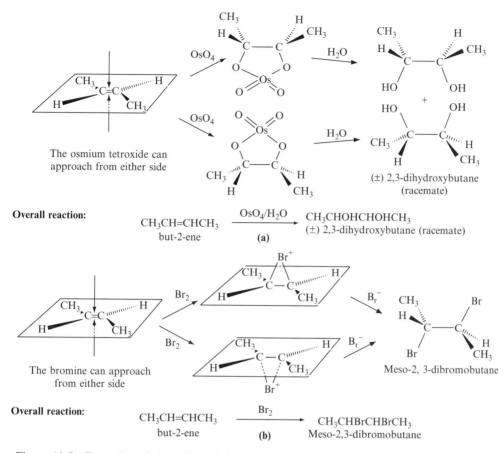

Figure 10.5 Examples of the effect of the nature of a reagent on the stereochemistry of a reaction. In both examples the reagent has an equal chance of attacking the C = C from either side

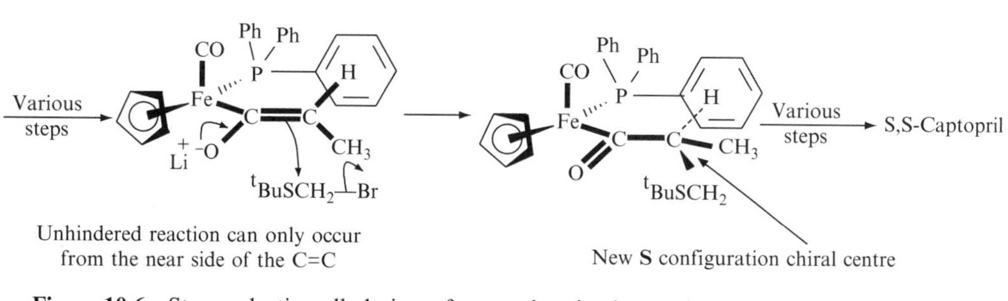

Figure 10.6 Stereoselective alkylation of an enolate in the synthesis of captopril. The heavier straight lines are bonds in the plane of the paper while the thin straight lines, are bonds behind the plane of the paper. The shape of the substrate means that an unhindered approach of the tertiary butylthiomethyl bromide (^{t}BuSCH$_2$Br) is only possible from one side of the iron-complex substrate. Consequently, reaction occurs mainly from this side of the complex, which results mainly in a product with an S configuration

discussed under the broad headings of either reactions that require a catalyst or those that do not require a catalyst for their stereoselectivity. However, it is emphasized that this and the subdivisions used are a simplification, and many reactions can fall into more than one category.

Methods that use catalysts to obtain stereoselectivity

Both enzyme (Figure 10.7) and non-enzyme catalysts (Figure 10.8) may be used.

A wide variety of enzyme controlled stereospecific transformations are known. These transformations include oxidations, reductions, reductive amina-tions, addition of ammonia, transaminations and hydrations. In each case the configuration of the new asymmetric centre will depend on the structure of the substrate. However, substrates whose reactive centres have similar structures will often produce asymmetric centres with the same configuration. Enzyme based methods are economical in their use of chiral material but suffer from the disadvantage that they can require large quantities of the enzyme to produce significant quantities of the drug.

A number of stereospecific non-enzyme catalysts have been developed that convert achiral substrates into chiral products. These catalysts are usually either complex organic (Figure 10.8(a)) or organometallic com-pounds (Figure 10.8(b)). The organometallic catalysts are usually optically active complexes whose structures usually contain one or more chiral ligands. An exception is the Sharpless–Katsuki epoxidation, which uses a mixture of an achiral titanium complex and an enantiomer of diethyl tartrate (Figure 10.8(c)).

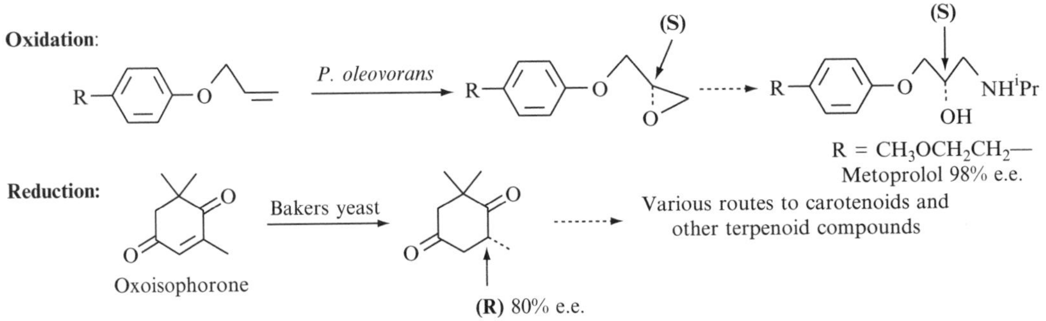

Figure 10.7   Examples of enzyme controlled transformations

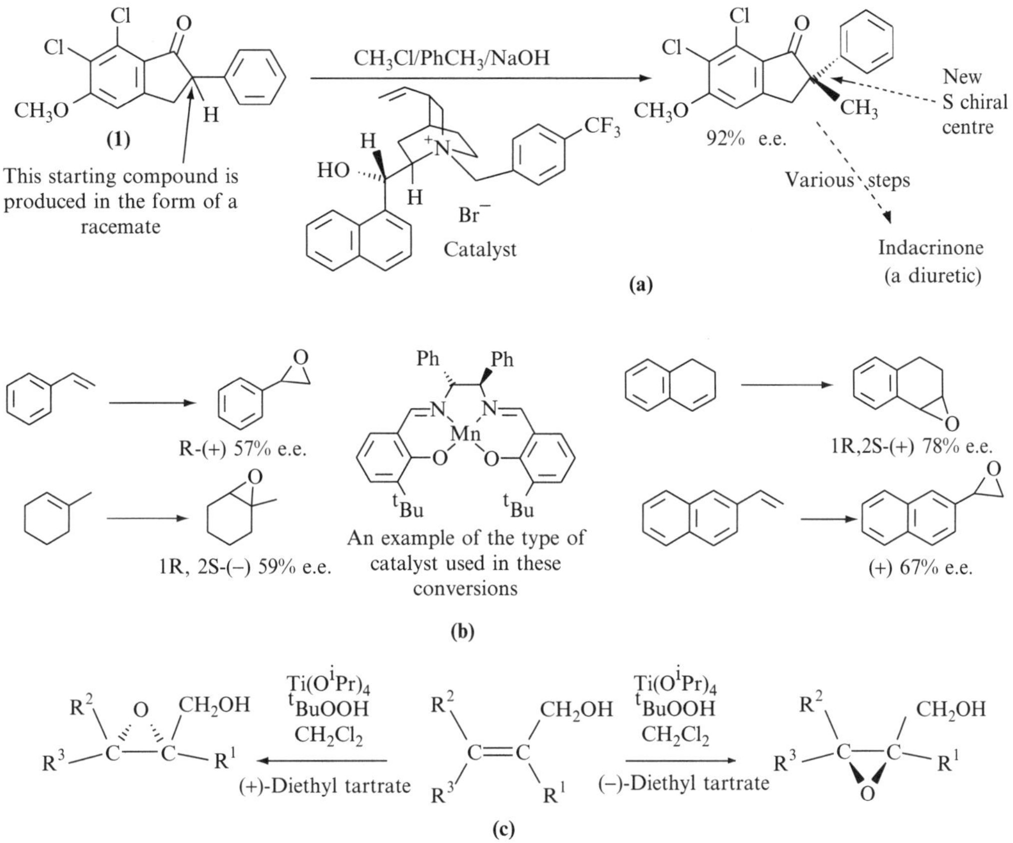

Figure 10.8 Examples of non-enzyme catalysed steroselective reactions with (a) a non-organometallic catalyst, (b) an organometallic catalyst and (c) a Sharpless–Katsuki catalyst

Methods that do not use catalysts to produce stereoselectivity

These general approaches can be classified for convenience as:

1. using chiral building blocks,

2. using a chiral auxiliary and

3. using achiral substrates and reagents.

1. **Using chiral building blocks**. These methods depend on the use of building blocks with the required configurations. A chiral building block whose structure contains the required configuration is reacted with a suitable substrate to introduce the desired asymmetric centre into the product (Figure 10.9). The

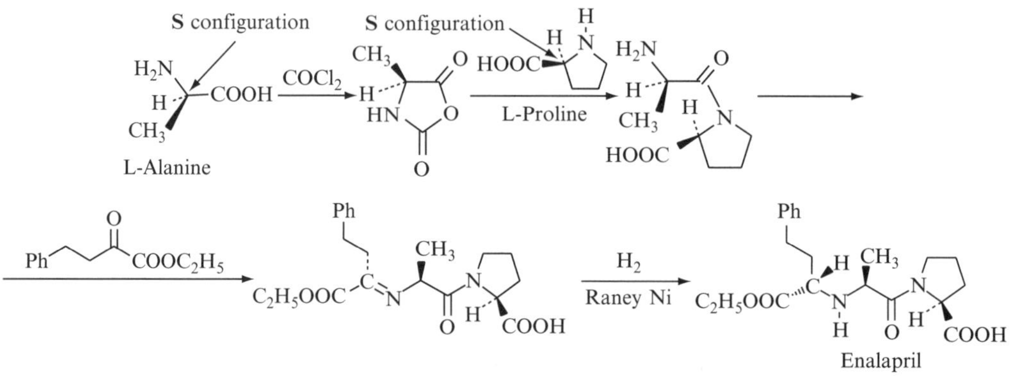

Figure 10.9 A synthetic route for the preparation of the ACE inhibitor enalapril (S-1-[N-(1-ethoxycarbonyl-3-phenylpropyl)-L-alanyl]-L-proline). The configurations of L-alanine and L-proline, the reagents for stage 2, are retained in the final product. The reduction of the intermediate A is stereoselective, giving the S,S,S-isomer in 87% yield

products of these types of reaction range from a single enantiomer to a mixture of diastereoisomers, which may be separated into their constituents (see section 10.2.1). In all cases, the reactions used in further stages of the synthesis should not affect the configurations of the chiral centres of the building blocks. However, in some instances reactions that cause an inversion of configuration may be used.

2. **Using a chiral auxiliary**. The achiral substrate is combined with a pure enantiomer known as a **chiral auxiliary** to form a chiral intermediate. Treatment of this intermediate with a suitable reagent produces the new asymmetric centre. The chiral auxiliary causes, by steric or other means (see section 10.2.2), the reaction to favour the production of one of the possible stereoisomers in preference to the others. Completion of the reaction is followed by removal of the chiral auxiliary, which may be recovered and recycled, thereby cutting down development costs (Figure 10.10). An advantage of this approach is that where the reaction used to produce the new asymmetric centre has a poor stereoselectivity the two products of the reaction will be diastereoisomers, as they contain two different asymmetric centres. These diastereoisomers may be separated by crystallization or chromatography (see section 10.2.1) and the unwanted isomer discarded.

3. **Using achiral substrates and reagents**. A wide variety of achiral substrates and reagents can give rise to asymmetric centres. For example, electrophilic addition of hydrogen chloride to butene gives rise to a racemic mixture of

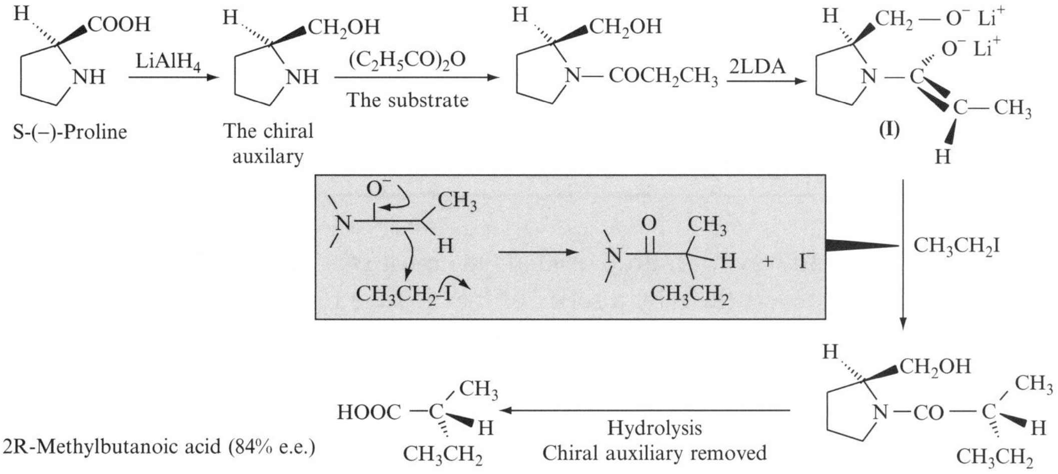

Figure 10.10 The synthesis of 2R-methylbutanoic acid, illustrating the use of a chiral auxiliary. The chiral auxiliary is 2S-hydroxymethyltetrahydropyrrole, which is readily prepared from the naturally occurring amino acid proline. The chiral auxiliary is reacted with propanoic acid anhydride to form the corresponding amide. Treatment of the amide with lithium diisopropylamide (LDA) forms the corresponding enolate (I). The reaction almost exclusively forms the Z-isomer of the enolate, in which the OLi units are well separated and possibly have the configuration shown. The approach of the ethyl iodide is sterically hindered from the top (by the OLi units or Hs) and so alkylation from the lower side of the molecule is preferred. Electrophilic addition to the appropriate enolate is a widely used method for producing the enantiomers of α-alkyl substituted carboxylic acids

the R and S isomers of 2-bromobutane because addition has an equal chance of occurring from either side of the $C = C$ bond.

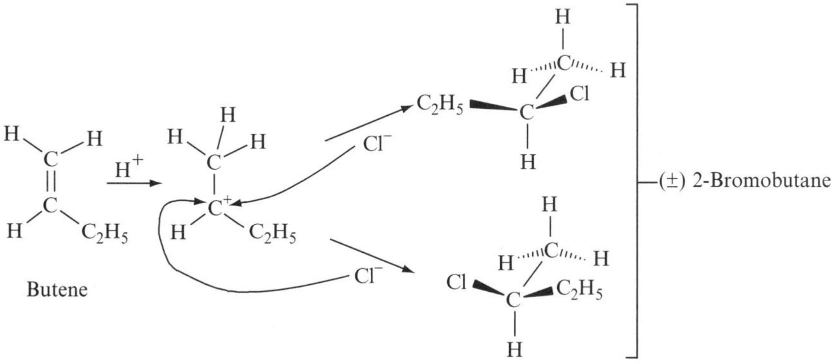

The usefulness of these reactions in stereoselective synthesis will depend on the nature of the product. If, for example, mixtures of enantiomers or diastereoisomers are formed, the usefulness of the reaction will also depend on the ease of separation of these mixtures into their component isomers.

10.3   Designing organic syntheses

The synthetic pathway for a drug or analogue must start with readily available materials and convert them by a series of inexpensive reactions into the target compound. There are no obvious routes as each compound will present a different challenge. The usual approach is to work back from the target structure in a series of steps until cheap commercially available materials are found. This approach is formalized by a method developed by S Warren, which is known as either the **disconnection approach** or **retrosynthetic analysis**. In all cases the final pathway should contain a minimum of stages, in order to keep costs to a minimum and overall yields to a maximum.

10.3.1   An introduction to the disconnection approach

This approach starts with the target structure and then works **backwards** by artificially cutting the target structure into sections known as **synthons**. Each of these backward steps is represented by a double shafted arrow ($\Longrightarrow$) whilst ⌇ is drawn through the disconnected bond of the target structure. Each of the possible synthons is converted on paper into a real compound known as a **reagent**, whose structure is similar to that of the synthon. All the possible disconnection routes must be considered. The disconnection selected for a step in the pathway is the one that gives rise to the best reagents for a reconnection reaction. This analysis is repeated with the reagents of each disconnection step until readily available starting materials are obtained. The selection of the reagents and the reactions for their reconnection may require extensive literature searches (Table 10.2).

   In the disconnection approach, bonds are usually disconnected by either homolytic or heterolytic fission (Figure 10.11(a) and (b)). However, some bonds may be disconnected by a reverse pericyclic mechanism (Figure 10.11(c)).

   Disconnections may involve either the carbon skeleton or functional groups. Normally the first step is to disconnect the sections of a molecule that are held together by functional groups such as esters, amides and acetals, as it is usually easier to find reconnection reactions for these functional groups. Heterolytic disconnections usually provide the most useful approach to synthesis design.

Table 10.2 Examples of books and databases that catalogue chemical reactions

Title	Author	Classification used
Books:		
Synthetic Organic Chemistry	Wagner and Zook	Lists reactions according to the functional group being produced.
Organic Functional Group Preparations.	Sandler and Karo	Lists reactions according to the functional group being produced.
Oxidations in Organic Chemistry	Hudlicky	Lists and discusses transformations that can be brought about by oxidation.
Reduction in Organic Chemistry	Hudlicky	Lists and discusses transformations that can be brought about by reduction.
Databases:		
CASREACT	The Chemical Abstracts Research Service	Information from 1985. Covers single and multistep reactions. Includes CAS Registry numbers of reactants, products, reagents, catalysts and solvents. It is structure searchable.
ISI Reaction Centre	Institute for Scientific Information	Data from 1840. Classified according to reaction type. Includes biological assays.
Crossfire	Beilstein Information Service	Three main types of data, structural and properties, reactions including preparations and chemical literature references.

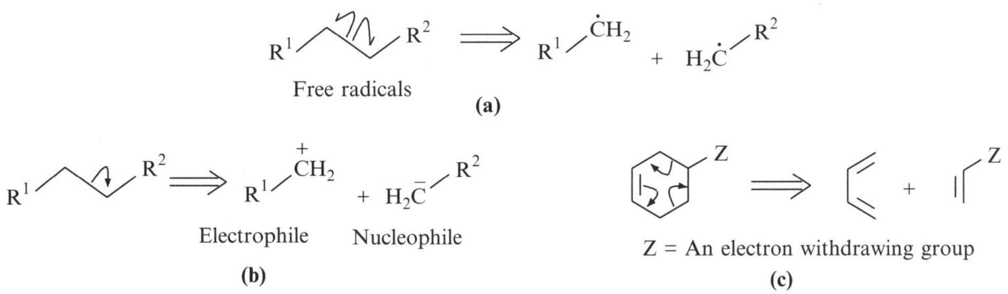

Figure 10.11 (a) Homolytic, (b) heterolytic and (c) pericyclic bond disconnections. Homolytic disconnections are usually disregarded because it is difficult to predict the outcome of reconnection reactions

This is because they divide the molecule into electrophilic and nucleophilic species, which can be more easily converted into the appropriate electrophilic and nucleophilic reagents for reconnection. The most useful heterolytic disconnections are those that give rise to either a stable species or occur by a feasible disconnection mechanism, such as hydrolysis, because the latter are more likely to have a corresponding reconnection reaction. At each stage in the disconnection, the synthons are used as a guide to selecting a corresponding real reagent that could be used in a reconversion synthesis. These reasgents are often compounds that possess the relevant electrophilic or nucleophilic reaction centres. For example, a carbanion synthon with the structure RCH_2^- could correspond to a Grignard reagent RCH_2MgBr. Similarly, an electrophilic synthon R^+CO could correspond to an acid halide $RCOCl$ or ester $RCOOR'$.

The basics of the technique of disconnection is illustrated by considering the synthesis of the local anaesthetic benzocaine. The most appropriate disconnections are the ester and amine groups. At this point it is a **matter of experience** as to which disassembly route is followed. The normal approach is to pick the synthons that give rise to reagents that can most easily be reformed into the product. Consequently, in this case the ester disconnection would appear to be the most profitable pathway, as ester formation is relatively easy, but it is notpossible to directly introduce a nucleophilic amino group into a benzene ring.

Benzocaine

4-Aminobenzoic acid

Key:

$|||$ = Indicates the real compound (derived from the synthon) that is used in the reconnection reaction.

Ethanol is a readily available starting material but 4-aminobenzoic acid is not. Therefore, the next step is to consider the disconnection of the amino and carboxylic acid groups of 4-aminobenzoic acid. However, there are no simple inexpensive reactions for the reconnection of these groups. Consequently, the next step has to be a **functional group interconversion** (FGI). Disconnection arrows are usually used for FGIs but as no synthons are involved it is customary to use real structures in the relationships. FGIs are found by searching the literature for suitable reactions. This search, in the case of the current example, reveals that aromatic carboxylic acids may be produced by the oxidation of anaromatic methyl group whilst an aromatic amine may be produced by reduction of the corresponding nitro group. Since amino groups are sensitive to oxidation the disconnection via functional group interconversion follows the order.

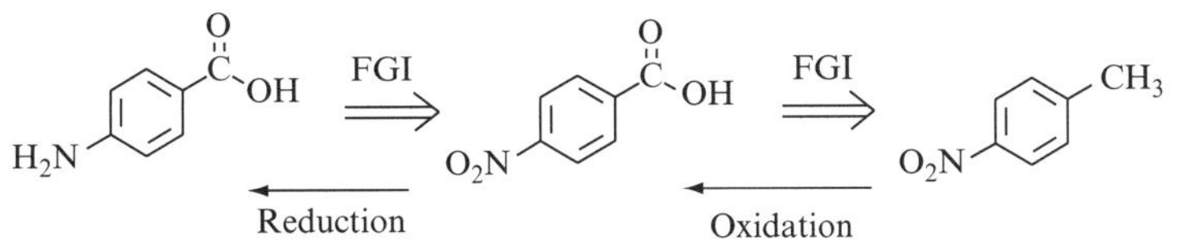

The retrosynthetic scheme (top):

4-aminobenzoic acid $\xrightarrow{\text{FGI}}$ 4-nitrobenzoic acid $\xrightarrow{\text{FGI}}$ 4-nitrotoluene

with the forward arrows labelled **Reduction** and **Oxidation** respectively.

The final stage is to consider the disconnection of both the methyl and nitro groups.

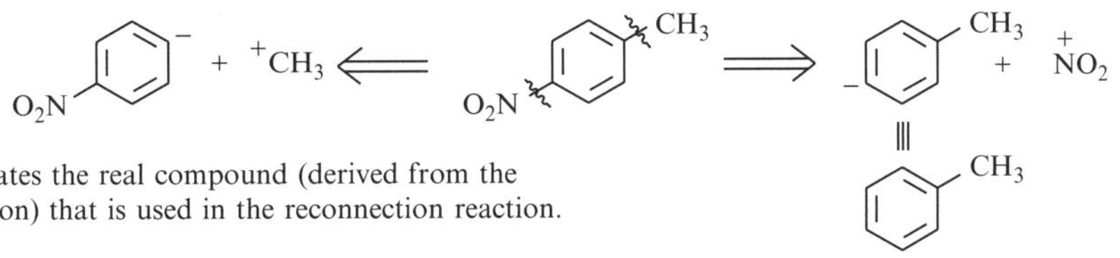

Disconnection scheme:

$$4\text{-nitro-}C_6H_4^- + {}^+CH_3 \Longleftarrow 4\text{-nitrotoluene} \Longrightarrow C_6H_5^- + CH_3\text{ (ring)} + {}^+NO_2$$

with toluene ($C_6H_5CH_3$) shown as the real compound.

Key:

$\parallel\!\parallel\!\parallel\ =$ Indicates the real compound (derived from the synthon) that is used in the reconnection reaction.

Toluene is a readily available compound, so the best disconnection is the nitro group. This is also supported by the fact that it is easy to form 4-nitrotoluene by nitration of toluene. Consequently, the complete synthesis is

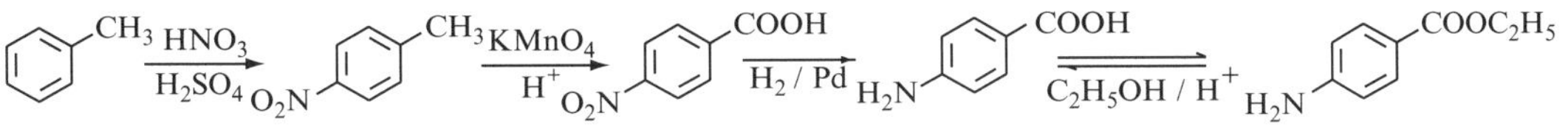

$$\text{toluene} \xrightarrow[\text{H}_2\text{SO}_4]{\text{HNO}_3} \text{4-nitrotoluene} \xrightarrow[\text{H}^+]{\text{KMnO}_4} \text{4-nitrobenzoic acid} \xrightarrow[\text{H}_2\text{N}]{\text{H}_2/\text{Pd}} \text{4-aminobenzoic acid} \xrightleftharpoons[\text{H}_2\text{N}]{\text{C}_2\text{H}_5\text{OH / H}^+} \text{ethyl 4-aminobenzoate}$$

The disconnection approach may be used for both linear and convergent syntheses (see section 10.2). However, in both cases the design of a synthesis using the approach must take into account the following:

1. the order of disconnection could influence the ease and direction of subsequent reactions;

2. the need to protect a reactive group in a compound by the use of a suitable protecting agent and

3. the need to incorporate chiral centres into the structure (see section 10.2.3).

A wide range of disconnections linked to suitable reconnections are known (Table 10.3). However, a number of functional groups are usually best introduced by FGI (Table 10.4). Once again it cannot be over-emphasized that their use will depend on the experience of the designer, which only improves with usage and time.

Table 10.3 Examples of most useful disconnections and reconnection systems. The compounds used for the reconnection reactions are those normally associated with the synthons for the disconnection. These reactions are not the only reactions that could be used for the reconnection. Source: *Organic Synthesis, the Disconnection Approach*, S Warren, Wiley. 1982

Disconnections	Examples of reconnection reactions

Functional group disconnections:

Ether:

$$R^1\text{-O}\!\!\!\!\text{-}R^2 \implies R^1\text{---}O^- + {}^+R^2$$

$$R^1\text{-OH} \xrightarrow{\text{Na}} R^1\text{---}O^-\ Na^+ \xrightarrow{R^2\text{-I}} R^1\text{---}O\text{---}R^2$$

Source of the nucleophile   Source of the electrophile

For methyl ethers use dimethyl sulphate instead of R^2I

Amide:

$$R^1NH\!\!\!\!\text{-}COR^2 \implies R^1\text{---}\bar{N}H + R^2\!\!-\overset{\overset{\displaystyle O}{\|}}{C}+$$

All types   Suitable acid
of amines   derivatives

$$R^1NH_2 + R^2COCl \longrightarrow R^1NH\text{---}COR^2$$

Source of the   Source of the
nucleophile   electrophile

Note: The acid anhydride will give the same compound but by a less vigorous reaction.

Ester:

$$R^1CO\!\!\!\!\text{-}OR^2 \implies R^1\!\!-\overset{\overset{\displaystyle O}{\|}}{C}+ \ + \ R^2\text{---}O^-$$

Suitable acid   All types of
derivatives   alcohol and phenol

$$R^1COCl + R^2OH \longrightarrow R^1CO\text{-}OR^2$$

Source of the   Source of the
electrophile   nucleophile

Note: The acid anhydride will give the same compound but by a less vigorous reaction.

Lactone:

$$\text{(ring)}\overset{O}{\underset{}{}}CO \implies \text{(ring)}\overset{O^-}{\underset{}{}}{}^+C=O$$

$$\text{(ring) OH, COOH} \xrightarrow{H^+} \text{(ring)}\overset{O}{\underset{}{}}CO$$

Source of both the nucleophile and electrophile

Carbon–carbon disconnections:

Carbanion–electrophile disconnections: Disconnection should normally occur adjacent to an electron withdrawing group. In each case, one of the compounds derived from the synthon should be able to form a carbanion whilst the structure of other should contain an electrophilic centre. Reconnection is by means of a suitable carbanion substitution or condensation reaction.

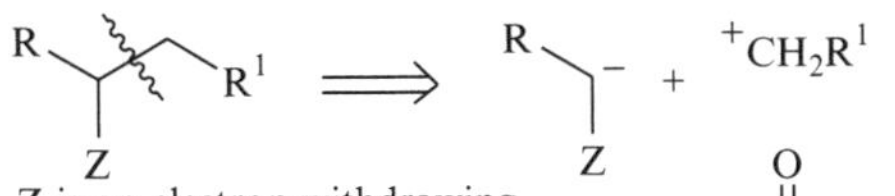

Z is an electron withdrawing
group, eg. NO_2, COOR, SOR,
SO_2R, CN.

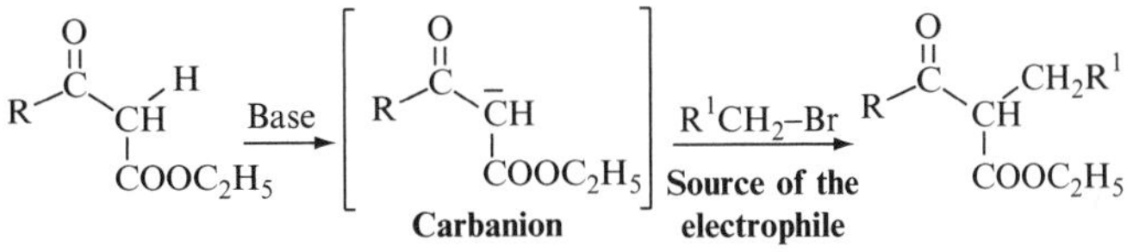

Carbanion **Source of the electrophile**

Friedel-Crafts disconnections:

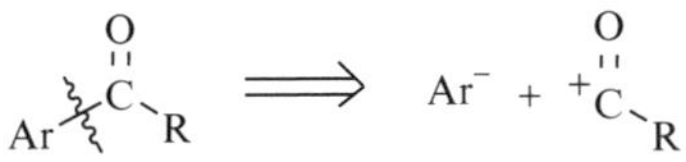

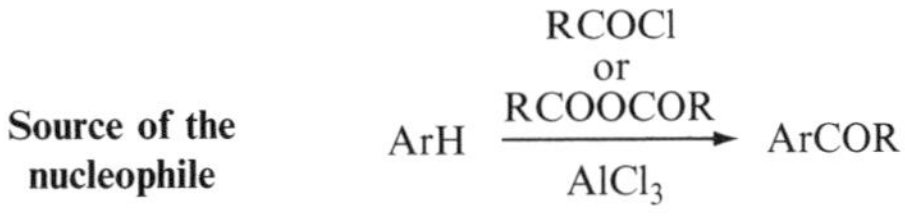

Source of the nucleophile

Ar = an aromatic system.

$$ArH \xrightarrow[AlCl_3]{\substack{RCOCl \\ or \\ RCOOCOR}} ArCOR$$

The position of substitution will depend on the nature of the
substituents on the aromatic (Ar) ring system

Adjacent to a ketone:

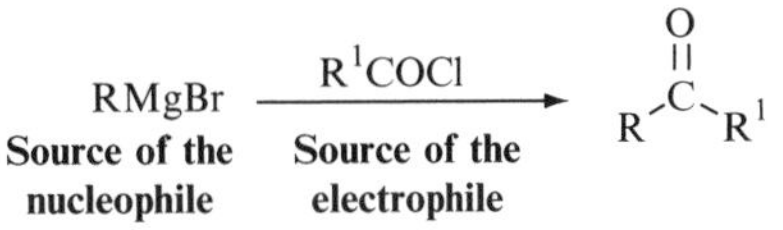

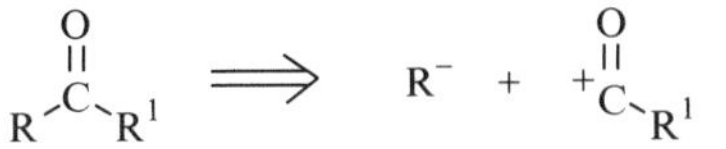

Source of the nucleophile **Source of the electrophile**

Adjacent to an alcohol:

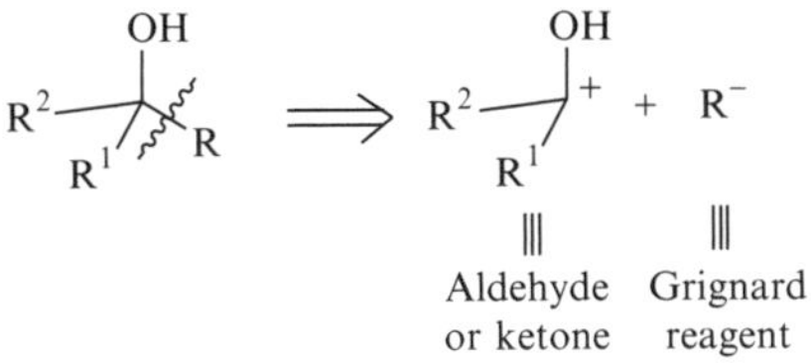

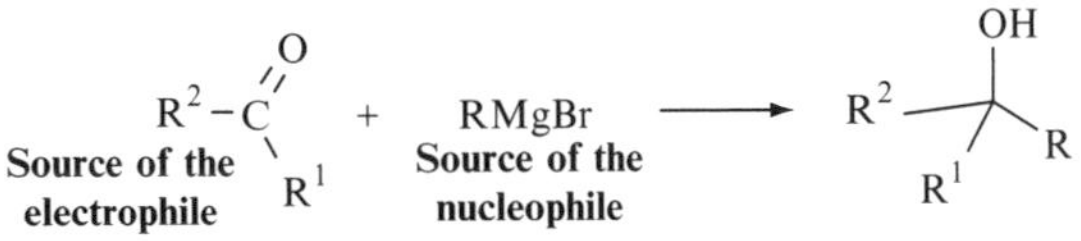

Aldehyde Grignard
or ketone reagent

Source of the electrophile **Source of the nucleophile**

Carboxylic acids:

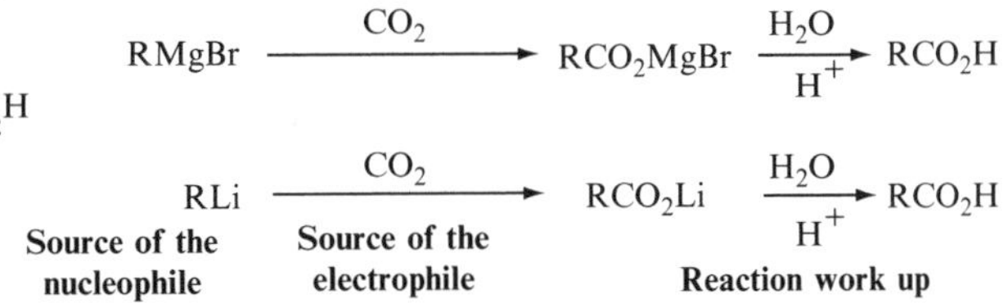

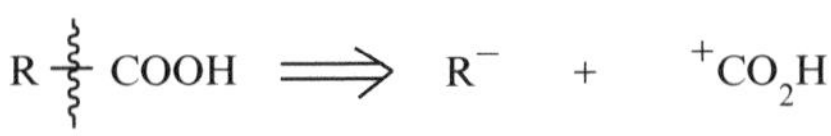

$R \rightleftharpoons COOH \implies R^- + {}^+CO_2H$

$$RMgBr \xrightarrow{CO_2} RCO_2MgBr \xrightarrow[H^+]{H_2O} RCO_2H$$

$$RLi \xrightarrow{CO_2} RCO_2Li \xrightarrow[H^+]{H_2O} RCO_2H$$

Source of the nucleophile **Source of the electrophile** **Reaction work up**

Table 10.4   Examples of reactions used to reverse FGIs. R can be both an aromatic and an aliphatic residue but Ar is only an aromatic residue

---

Alkenes: By elimination of alcohols and halides.

Aldehydes and ketones: By oxidation of the appropriate alcohol.

$$RCH_2OH \xrightarrow{\text{Oxidation}} RCHO$$

Primary alcohol   Aldehyde

$$\begin{array}{c} R \\ {}_{R^1} \end{array}\!CH{-}OH \xrightarrow{\text{Oxidation}} \begin{array}{c} R \\ {}_{R^1} \end{array}\!C{=}O$$

Secondary alcohol   Ketone

Amines:

$$R{-}NO_2 \xrightarrow{\text{Reduction}} R{-}NH_2$$

$$RCONHR^1 \xrightarrow{\text{Reduction}} RCH_2NHR^1$$

Useful one carbon additions to aromatic ring systems:

$$Ar{-}H \xrightarrow[\text{Chloromethylation}]{\text{HCHO/HCl/ZnCl}_2} Ar{-}CH_2Cl$$

$$Ar{-}OH \xrightarrow[\text{Riemer-Tiemann}]{\text{CHCl}_3\text{/OH}^-} Ar\!\begin{array}{c} \nearrow OH \\ \searrow CHO \end{array}$$

Phenols

10.4   Questions

---

(1) Explain the meaning of the terms (i) linear, (ii) convergent and (iii) partial synthetic pathways.

(2) Outline the practical considerations that need to be taken into account when selecting reactions for use in a synthetic pathway.

(3) Describe the use of catalysts in asymmetric synthesis.

(4) What is a chiral auxiliary? Suggest a feasible stereospecific synthesis for 2R-methylhexanoic acid starting from S-(−)-proline and propanoic anhydride.

(*continued*)

(5) Explain the meaning of the term 'synthon'. Draw the best synthons and their corresponding real compounds for each of the following compounds:

(i)

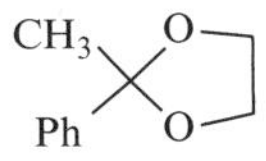

(ii)

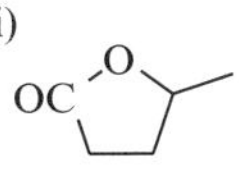

(iii)

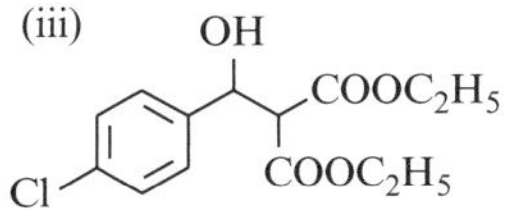

(iv)

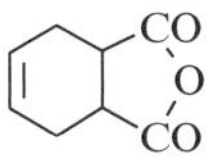

(6) What is the significance of the initials FGI in the disconnection approach to designing synthetic pathways? Suggest the best disconnection sequences for the synthesis of each of the following compounds:

(i)

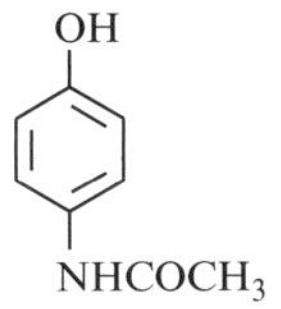

(ii)

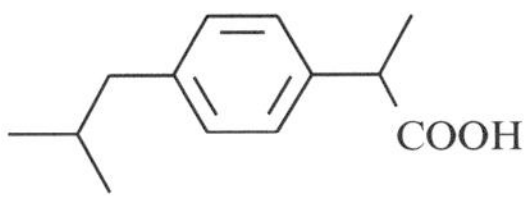

11 Drug Development and Production

11.1 Introduction

Development is the conversion of a biologically active compound into a safe marketable product. It is a multi-disciplinary process, which requires the collaboration of teams of workers from many different disciplines. Its success is dependent on their skills and judgement. This chapter will outline the work carried out by these teams in the main areas of the development process. The activities in many of these areas are interdependent, which means that they should take place consecutively or at the same time. Consequently, as speed is of the essence in all development work, these activities will require careful planning and coordination.

The development process normally takes between seven and ten years from initiation to marketing the drug. Furthermore, only one in 400–1000 drug candidates considered for development ever reach the market. Consequently, development is very expensive, the average cost of successfully developing a drug being estimated to be about 350 million pounds in 1999. As a result, the high risk nature of development means that it is necessary to plan a comprehensive strategy to reduce both the pharmaceutical and financial risks. The first step in this strategy is to define product pharmaceutical and financial targets and assess whether the drug will reach these goals. Consequently, it is essential to assess whether the new drug will be able to compete with existing competitors and what advantages it may have over those competitors. This assessment should be repeated at appropriate points in the development to ensure that the development is still viable. The management of this and other aspects of the development is often performed by monitoring its **critical path** (Figure 11.1). This consists of the activities that determine the time taken for the drug to

Fundamentals of Medicinal Chemistry, Edited by Gareth Thomas
© 2003 John Wiley & Sons, Ltd
ISBN 0 470 84306 3 (Hbk), ISBN 0 470 84307 1 (pbk)

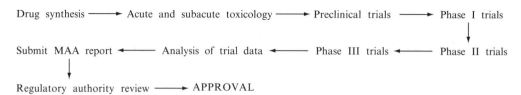

Figure 11.1 An example of the activities that are likely to form the critical path for the development of a drug. MAA is the market authorization application that a company has to submit in Britain in order to produce and market a drug

become registered by the appropriate government body. It does not include all the activities that are necessary to to develop and evaluate a drug. However, monitoring the critical path does provide a way of making certain the project remains on schedule.

11.2   Chemical development

The reactions used by research workers frequently use expensive reagents and only produce sufficient quantities of the drug for very limited biological testing. In addition, the research routes often involve techniques, such as chromatography, that cannot be adapted to large scale production methods. Consequently, the **first** step in the chemical synthesis development is to find safe, cost effective alternatives. These alternative reactions should start from cheap readily available materials, consist of more economical reactions that have high yields and be capable of being safely carried out on a large laboratory or manufacturing scale (see section 11.2.4). They should yield sufficient quantities of the lead in an acceptable purity for the initial activity and toxicology tests. Initially several large scale synthetic routes will be investigated in order to determine the optimum route. Convergent routes are usually preferred over linear syntheses as they give better overall yields (see section 10.2). However, in the early stages of development, speed of production of sufficient amounts of the lead for comprehensive testing is often more important than devising a chemically efficient synthesis. This is because the results of these initial tests will enable the company managers to decide whether the compound is worth further development.

The progression of the drug through the development process will lead to an increased demand for larger quantities of the drug. This demand is normally met by conversion of the most promising laboratory synthesis to pilot plant scale. Conversion of a synthesis to pilot plant scale, which is effectively a mini-manufacturing process, may require changes in the synthesis to allow for the use of large scale equipment (see section 11.2.1). These changes, waste disposal and the hazards associated with carrying out the synthesis using larger amounts of the reagents should be evaluated before the conversion is made (see section 11.2.2). The pilot plant should produce sufficient quantities of the drug to carry out the comprehensive tests that are required by the regulating authority. Once a licence to manufacture the drug has been granted, the pilot plant synthesis is converted to the full manufacturing process. The main considerations in this conversion are chemical engineering issues, environmental impact, waste disposal, safety, quality control and cost.

11.2.1 Chemical engineering issues

Initially, the chemical engineers will have to decide whether the reactions can be safely carried out in the existing plant or whether it will be necessary to construct a new plant. Since the latter could be very expensive, they should also consider whether it is possible to modify the synthesis so that it could utilize existing equipment. The standard large scale reaction vessel is a stainless steel container. It is usually equipped with a stirring paddle, a heating jacket for controlling the reaction temperature, openings that allow solids and liquids to be placed in or removed from the vessel and provision for either distilling or refluxing liquids (Figure 11.2). Reaction vessels are usually connected by

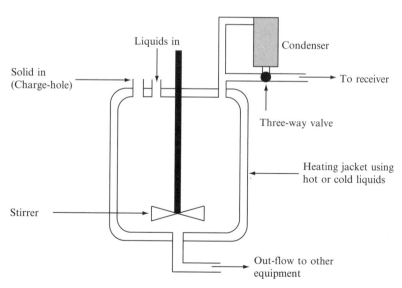

Figure 11.2 A diagramatic representation of a typical reaction vessel. The three way valve enables the condenser to be used to either reflux or distil the liquids in the reaction vessel

suitable pipework to other pieces of specialized plant such as filtration, crystal-lization and drying equipment. A variety of methods are used to transfer the product from the reaction vessel to these additional pieces of equipment. They include the use of pumps, nitrogen gas under pressure, screw and conveyor systems. Separations are usually carried out using the reaction vessel as the separator and running the lower liquid phase out of the bottom of the reaction vessel. Control of the reaction and, if required, a subsequent operations are achieved by the use of appropriate sensor systems and small armoured glass windows known as sight-glasses, which enable the plant operators to view the contents of the vessel and/or pipework.

The reactions selected for pilot and manufacturing processes must take into account the limitations of the available plant, for example the reaction vessel and the ancillary equipment required for isolation and purification of the product. Reaction vessels usually have an operating range of between about -15 and about $+140°C$. Consequently, as both heating and cooling are expen-sive, the reactions selected should give a satisfactory yield as near to room temperature as possible and certainly within the temperature control limits of the vessel. Furthermore, large scale reactions require longer processing times, because they take longer to reach their working temperature, produce a satis-factory yield and cool down than laboratory preparations. This means that the reagents, products, solvents and catalysts used must have an adequate degree of stability under the prevailing operating conditions.

11.2.2 Chemical plant, health and safety considerations

Health and safety is of paramount importance when selecting the reactions for either the pilot or manufacturing processes. A full chemical hazard assess-ment should be carried out before commencing the reaction on a large scale. This should cover the chemistry of the process, the safety of the plant operatives, waste disposal and its impact on the environment. The chemical and biological hazards associated with all the chemicals and solvents used in the reactions should be documented, together with protocols for dealing with accidents, leaks and spillages. Even in the best regulated chemical plants there will be some leakage of compounds, such as solvent vapour and chemical dust into the atmosphere, and so monitoring equipment must be appropriate for the sub-stances being used. Reactions that involve handling highly toxic substances should not be used unless there is no alternative. In this case a stringent protocol governing their use must be drawn up and enforced. One important consider-ation for all health and safety protocols is the nature of the thermochemistry of the reactions. The heat generated by a large scale reaction may exceed the cooling capacity of the existing equipment with disastrous results. Consequently, if they are not known, the heats of reaction for each of the stages used in the process must be accurately determined and taken into account when assessing the safety of the plant and its operatives.

Waste disposal and its environmental impact are becoming increasingly important and must now be planned for as part of the development process. In the past, solid wastes were buried in special landfill sites but now because of potential water pollution it is regarded as undesirable unless alternative methods, such as incineration, are not suitable. Aqueous liquids may be discharged into the sewage system, rivers and the sea. However, this requires removal of high concentrations of impurities, especially metals, such as copper, zinc, mercury and cadmium, and organic halogen compounds, such as chloroform, which are highly toxic to many forms of aquatic life. Solvents are usually recovered by distillation but this is not always a practical proposition for some solvents such as dimethyl sulphoxide and N,N-dimethylformamide. Gases can often be prevented from entering the atmosphere by reaction with suitable absorbents in absorbent towers. However, gases such as nitric oxide that cannot be disposed of in this manner require special treatment, which can be very expensive. In all cases the disposal of highly toxic waste is to be avoided, as it can require expensive special treatment.

An idea of the impact of a process on the environment may be determined from its effluent load factor (ELF). This is defined as

$$\mathrm{ELF} = \frac{\text{mass of all ingredients of all the stages} - \text{mass of the product}}{\text{mass of the product}} \quad (11.1)$$

The ELF is the amount of waste produced by the process per unit mass of the product. It can refer to individual stages in the synthesis or the whole process. In the ideal situation, where all the ingredients are converted into the product, the ELF value will be zero. This does not happen in synthetic processes. In pharmaceutical processes, the ELF is usually of the order of 100. The process design chemists will aim to minimize the ELF in order to reduce expense by selection of the reactions and the operation of the plant.

11.2.3 Synthesis quality control

The efficiency of drug production will depend on being able to identify and assess the chemical purity of the drug and also that of the intermediate compounds involved at each step in the synthesis. This means that it is normally necessary to devise appropriate chemical quantitative and qualitative protocols for all of the compounds involved in the pilot and manufacturing routes. Physical methods, such as HPLC and GC, are often used for these purposes. It is also necessary to be able to identify impurities and any closely related structures or stereoisomers as this will be required by the licencing authority. Consequently, some thought should be given to how all these analyses may be made when designing the production route.

In some synthetic routes, an intermediate product may be used in the next stage of the synthesis without it being isolated and purified. This procedure is known as **telescoping**. It has the advantage of avoiding handling very toxic intermediates. It also makes it easier to deal with non-crystalline and oily products. In order for telescoping to be effective, the initial reaction has to produce a relatively pure product. Consequently, when this technique is used an analytical procedure must be available to ensure that the purity of the product is high enough for the next reaction to be carried out in an efficent manner.

11.2.4 A case study

Adapted from S. Lee and G. Robinson, *Process Development, Fine Chemicals from Grams to Kilograms*, Oxford University Press, 1995.

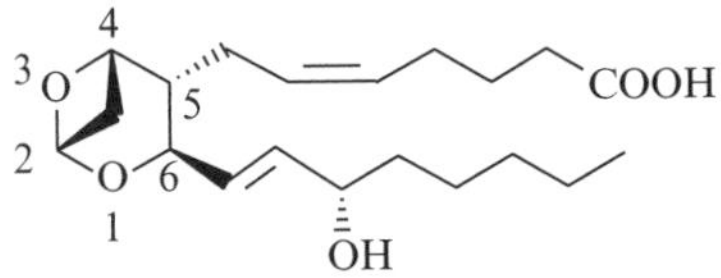

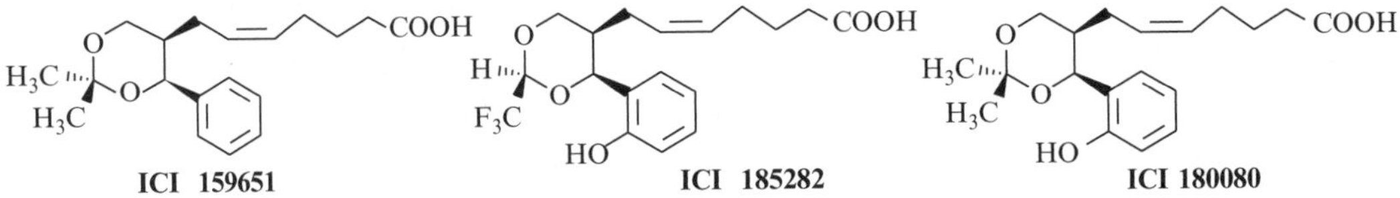

Figure 11.3 (a) Thromboxane A_2 (TXA$_2$). *Note:* The locants given are those of the dioxan ring only and not those for the complete molecule. They are used for reference purposes only (see text). (b) Examples of some of the thromboxane antagonists developed by ICI

The release of thromboxane A_2 (Figure 11.3(a)) in the body can cause a number of toxic reactions including bronchoconstriction, blood vessel constriction and platelet aggregation. This activity led ICI to develop a number of compounds that can act as antagonists for thromboxane (Figure 11.3(b)). It was found that significant antagonist activity is obtained when:

1. at position 2 there is a substituent *cis* to the other substituents of the dioxan ring,

2. the phenolic and alkenoic acid side chains at positions 5 and 6 have a *cis* orientation and

3. the C=C of the alkenoic acid side chain has a *cis* configuration.

These active analogues were initially synthesized in gram quantities by routes that allowed numerous analogues to be produced for the preliminary biological evaluation (Figure 11.4).

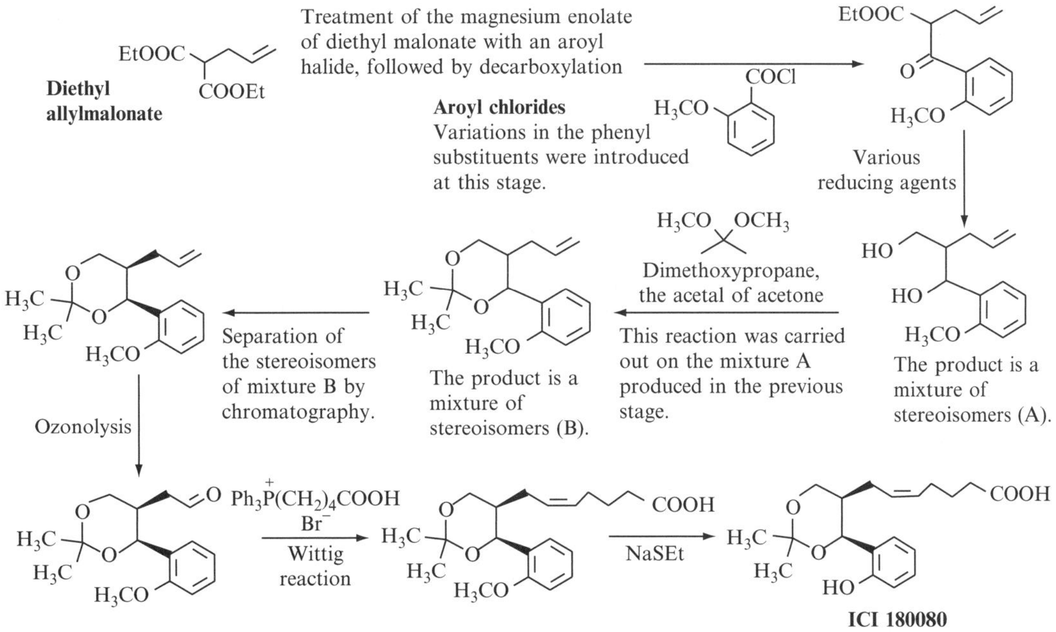

Figure 11.4 An outline of the initial research route for the synthesis of ICI 180080 and other analogues. The intermediates and products were produced as racemates. Geometric stereoisomers were synthesized as shown in the reaction scheme.

The potential manufacturing route for the active thromboxane antagonists synthesized by the small scale route outlined in Figure 11.4 must include a way of controlling the stereochemistry of the product that will also give a single enantiomer. In addition, it must also include alternatives to the chromatographic separation, since this technique is not practical on a large scale, the ozonolysis, which is very expensive and needs specialized equipment, and sodium ethanethiolate, which would need special containment since it is a volatile liquid with a vile odour.

The initial manufacturing scale route (Figure 11.5) used the formation of a suitably substituted 1,4-butrolactone by a Perkin reactions any phenolic hydroxyl groups were protected by forming their methyl ethers. The investigators found that the 3,4-substituents of these lactone ring should be *trans* to each other in order to produce a final product in which these substituents had the required *cis* orientation in the dioxan ring. The reduction of the lactone to the lactol enabled the team to use a Wittig reaction to introduce the *cis* alkenoic acid side chain into the structure. Although this reaction produces a mixture of isomers, it was relatively easy to isolate a relatively pure *cis* product. The use of the Wittig reaction also avoids the use of ozonolysis and the expense of specialized plant. Cyclization of the product from the Wittig reaction, achieved by a variety of routes, depending on the nature and stability of the final product, was

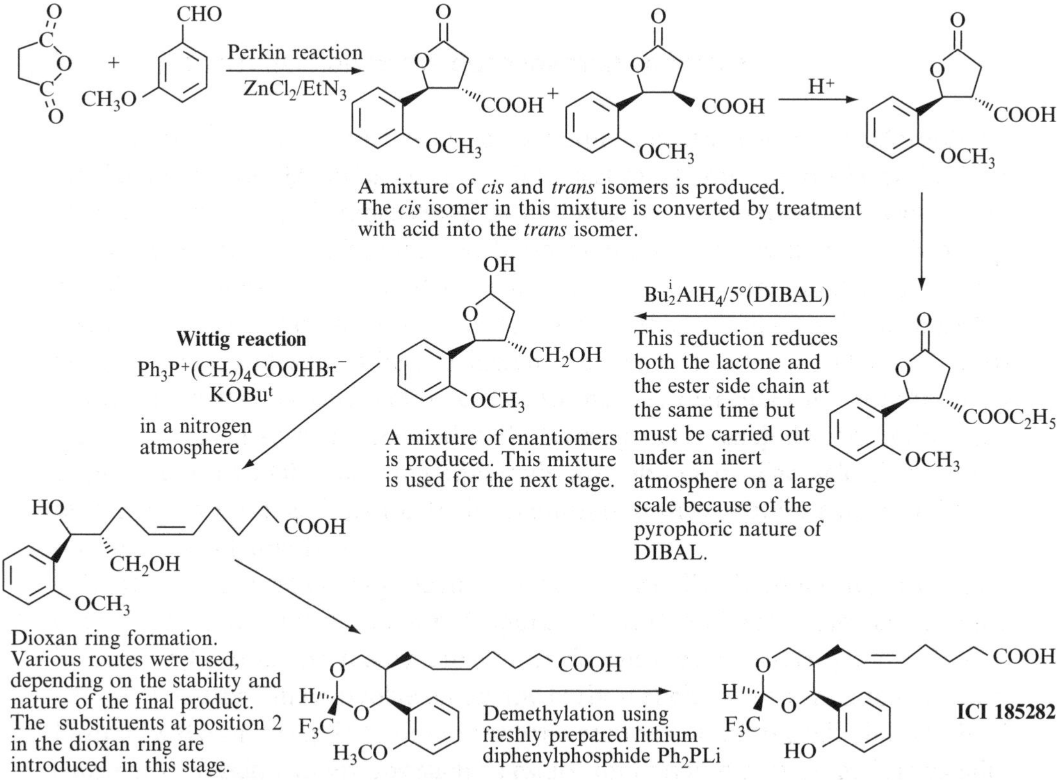

Figure 11.5 An outline of the manufacturing route developed for the production of ICI 185282 and its analogues. Both succinic anhydride and the appropriate aromatic aldehydes are readily available

used to form the dioxan ring. Finally, where appropriate, the use of sodium ethanethiolate to remove the methyl protecting groups of any phenolic hydroxy groups was avoided by the use of lithium diphenylphosphide. Demethylation was simply carried out by adding the methyl ether to freshly prepared lithium diphenylphosphide, which made this reaction highly suitable for large scale production methods. It was reported that using the route outlined in Figure 11.5, products containing less than 1% of stereoisomers were produced on an industrial scale.

11.3   Pharmacological and toxicological testing

Extensive pharmacological and toxicological testing must be carried out on any new drug before it is marketed. These tests are carried out in two stages, namely, **preclinical** and **clinical trials**. These trials assess the risks involved with the use of the new drug. They may also provide vital information concerning pharmaco-kinetic properties of the drug, which can be used in other areas of the development. Details of the trials are given in the MAA application which is submitted to the appropriate government body (see section 11.8). This body will either approve of the trials programme or specify modifications. To develop and market the drug, the producer must comply with all the terms of the MAA, which has replaced the older drug licience. It is essentially a scientific assessment of the safety, efficacy and quality of the new product.

Preclinical trials are essentially toxicity and other biological tests carried out by microbiologists on bacteria and pharmacologists on tissue samples, animals and sometimes organ cultures to determine whether it is safe to test the drug on humans. The animal tests investigate the effect of the drug on various body systems such as the respiratory, nervous and cardiovascular systems. They are carried out under both *in vivo* (in the living organism) and *in vitro* (in an artifical environment) conditions. These preliminary tests also provide other information concerning the drug's pharmacokinetic properties and its interaction with other drugs and over-the-counter medicines. If necessary, any of these interactions that enhance or reduce the drugs activity should be investigated further during the clinical trials and the results noted in the product labelling and literature.

The preclinical tests should help decide whether it is safe to give the the drug to humans and also the toxic dose for humans. This enables the investigators to set a dose level to start the Phase I clinical trials. These will include dose-ranging pharmacokinetic studies and bioavailability via chosen administration routes. However, relating animal tests to humans is difficult and the results are only acceptable if the dose–organ toxicity findings include a substantial safety margin.

The use of animals in drug testing is the subject of considerable debate in the pharmaceutical industry as well as by the general public. Most countries are committed to reducing the number of animals used in this way to a minimum and are actively investigating the use of chemical and other alternative methods. These methods include avoiding replication of experiments by different countries centralizing their validation procedures, using human cell *in vitro* tests instead of animal *in vivo* tests and eliminiating methods that are not relevant to humans. However, it is unlikely that it will be possible to replace all animal testing. Once the drug has passed the preclinical trials it undergoes clinical trials in humans. These trials can raise legal and ethical problems and so must be approved by the appropriate legal and ethical committees before the trials are conducted. In most countries this approval requires the issuing of a certificate or licence by the appropriate medicine control agency (see section 11.8).

In order to accurately assess the results of a clinical trial, the results must be compared with the normal situation and so, in the trials conducted on healthy humans, 50% of the subjects are normally given an inactive substance in a form that cannot be distinguished from the test substance. This inactive dosage form is known as a **placebo**. Furthermore, the results of a trial must be reliable and not subject to influence by either the person conducting the trial or the recipient of the drug. Consequently, it is now common practice to carry out a **double blind** procedure, where both the administrator of the drug and the recipient are unaware whether they are dealing with the drug itself or a placebo. In addition, subjects are randomly chosen to receive either the placebo or the drug.

Trials conducted on healthy subjects do not demonstrate the beneficial action of the new drug. It is necessary to carry out double blind trials on unhealthy patients to assess its efficacy. However, the use of a placebo with patients who are ill raises moral and ethical considerations. Placebos may still be used if the withdrawal of therapy causes no lasting harm to patients. If this is not possible, the effect of the new drug is compared with that of an established drug used to treat the medical condition. This reference drug should be carefully selected. It should not be chosen so as to give the new drug an inflated degree of potency that could be used to give the manufacturer an unfair commercial advantage and the patient an inaccurate idea of the medicine's effectiveness. A third alternative is to use **cross over** trials. Halfway through the trial the patients receiving the drug are switched to either the placebo or the reference drug and the patients receiving the placebo or reference drug are given the new drug. This is ethically more acceptable as both groups have been exposed to the benefits of the new drug.

The first clinical trials (**Phase I** trials) are usually conducted on small groups of healthy volunteers, which do not include children and the elderly. These volunteers undergo an exhaustive medical examination before the tests and are strictly monitored at all times during the trial. The trials are conducted in either in house-clinics or specialist outside facilities. The objective of these trials on healthy humans is to ascertain the behaviour of the new drug in the human body. They also yield information on the dosage form, absorption, distribution, bioavailability, elimination and side effects of the new drug. The relation of the side effects to specific metabolites allows medicinal chemists to eliminate the side effects by designing new analogues that do not give rise to that metabolite (see section 9.8.). In addition, the trials give information concerning the level of the drug in the blood after intravenous and oral dosing, rate of excretion in the urine and via the bowel and the effect of gender on these parameters. At all times in the trials the function of the kidney and other organs in the body are monitored for adverse reactions. The dose administered to the volunteers is initially a small fraction of that administered by the same route to animals.

Once the safety of the drug has been assessed in healthy volunteers the testing programme moves to **Phase II** trials. However, before these trials can be carried out in Britain the company must obtain a clinical trials certificate, which is issued by the regulating authority. Phase II trials are conducted on small numbers of patients with the condition that the drug has been designed to treat. They assess the drug's effectiveness in treating the condition and also help establish a dose level and dosage regimen for the drug. The success of this phase leads to **Phase III** trials, where the the new product is tried out on large numbers of patients. In Britain, Phase II trials may only be carried out after a local ethics committee has evaluated and approved the trials programme (see section 11.8). Phase III trials are carried out using both placebos and comparison standards. They are particulary useful for obtaining safety and efficacy data in order to satisfy the product licencing authorities. In both Phase II and III trials a few subjects will exhibit **adverse drug reactions** (ADRs). These are described as responses that are either unwanted or harmful, which occur at the doses used for therapy. They exclude therapy failure. These ADRs are noted and added to the drug's data sheet. However, unless a high percentage of subjects exhibit the same ADR they do not usually result in the drug being withdrawn from use.

When the new drug has been released onto the market the performance of the drug is monitored using very large numbers of patients both in hospital and general practice. This monitoring is often refered to as the **Phase IV** trials. It provides more information about the drug's safety and efficiacy. In addition trials are conducted on specific aspects of the drug's use with smaller specialist groups, for example, its kinetics in the elderly, infants, neonates and ethnic groups.

The interpretation of the results of all trials requires the close collaboration of clinicians and statisticians. Reliable results are only obtained if at least the minimum number of patients for statistical viability are involved in the preliminary trials. It is often difficult to measure precisely the parameter chosen for assessment. Consequently, results are usually quoted in terms of a probability coefficient, the lower the value of this coefficient the more accurate the results. However, very reliable results will only be obtained from clinical trials if large groups of patients are tested. This is seldom feasible. Consequently, manufacturers and licencing authorities usually settle for the best statistical compromise. Since some adverse effects do not manifest themselves for years, it is necessary to constantly monitor the drug (Phase IV trials) after it has been released for general use.

A more effective interpretation of pharmacological and toxicological data may usually be made if the ADMEs of the drug and its metabolites are well defined (see section 8.4). Tissue distribution data is usually obtained using single dose studies but repeated dose studies should be undertaken when:

1. the tissue $t_{1/2}$ of the drug or metabolite is much larger than its plasma $t_{1/2}$ value,

2. the C_{ss} of the drug or its metabolites is found to be very much higher than that predicted from single dose studies,

3. the drug is targeted at a specific site and

4. particular types of tissue show unexpected lesions.

11.4   Drug metabolism and pharmacokinetics

Drug metabolism and pharmacokinetic (DMPK) studies are used to show how the concentrations of the drug and its metabolites vary with the administered dose of the drug and the time from administration. They are normally carried out using suitable animal species and in humans in Phase I trials. The information obtained from animal studies is used to determine safe dose levels for use in the Phase I clinical trials in humans. However, the accuracy of the data obtained from animal tests is limited, since it is obtained by extrapolation. In addition, it is necessary to determine the dose that just saturates the absorption and elimination processes so that the toxicological and pharmacological events may be correctly interpreted.

11.5   Formulation development

The form in which a drug is administered to patients is known as its **dosage form**. Dosage forms can be subdivided according to their physical nature into liquid, semisolid and solid formulations. Liquid formulations include solutions, syrups, suspensions and emulsions. Creams, ointments and gels are normally regarded as semisolid formulations, whereas tablets, capsules, suppositories, pessaries and transdermal patches are classified as solid formulations. However, all these dosage forms consist of the drug and ingredients known as **excipients**. Excipients have a number of functions, such as fillers (bulk providing agents), lubricants, binders, preservatives and antioxidants. A change in the nature of the excipient can significantly affect the release of the drug from the dosage form. Consequently, manufacturers must carry out bioavailability and any other tests specified by the licencing authority if they make changes to the dosage form before marketing the new dosage form.

The type of dosage form required will depend on the nature of the target and the stage in the drug development. Since many promising drug candidates fail at the preclinical and Phase I stages, a simple dosage form, such as a oral solution, is often used for the preclinical and early Phase I clinical trials. This is in order to keep costs to a minimum at these high risk stages of drug development. However, the manufacturer must also use the dosage form of the drug that he proposes to use in the later clinical trials.

The types of dosage form used must satisfy criteria such as stability and pattern of drug release. Stability studies are used to determine whether the dosage form has an adequate potency after an appropriate period of time, usually 2–3 years. This will determine its shelf life and recommended storage conditions. Drug release is directly influenced by the excipients and any slow release mechanisms employed. In both these examples suitable chemical and biological experiments must be designed to either obtain or check the relevant data. The results of these experiments may lead to improvements in the design of the dosage form. They are usually carried out in parallel with the clinical trials.

11.6   Production and quality control

The manufacture of the new drug must be carried out under the conditions laid down in the marketing authorization (MA) (see section 11.8). Since it is not usually practical for manufacturers to dedicate a plant to the production of one particular drug, it is essential that the equipment used is cleaned and tested for adulterants before use. Many pharmaceutical manufacturers estimated that production line equipment is only used to produce the product for about 10% of its time. For most of the remaining time it is being stripped down, cleaned and reassembled.

The quality control of drugs and medicines during and after production is essential for their safe use. It was only achieved when accurate analytical methods were developed in the mid-19th century. This led to the publication of national pharmacopoeias and other documents that specified the extent and the nature of the identification tests and quantitative assessments required to ensure that the product reaching the public is fit for its purpose. These documents now cover the production, storage and application of pharmaceutical products. They are the subject of constant review but unfortunately this does not completely prevent the occurrence of product related problems. However, the continual updating of these documents does reduce the possibility of similar problems occurring in other products. It is gratifying to note that since the thalidomide disaster very few drugs have been removed from the market on safety grounds. The development of reliable analytical methods for the trials, production quality control and identification, limit and assay procedures for inclusion into the relevant pharmacopoeias is normally carried out in parallel to the critical path development stages. These analytical methods must be described in detail in the product licence application.

11.7 Patent protection

The high cost of drug development and production makes it essential for a company to maximize its returns from a new drug. This can only be achieved by preventing unrestricted copying of a new product by rivals. Patents are used to prevent rival companies manufacturing and marketing a product without the permission of the originator of the product. However, many companies do market other manufacturers' products under licence from the original patentor.

Patents have been used, in one form or another, as a means of industrial protection from the early 14th century to the present day. Originally, they were intended to encourage the development of new industries and products by granting the developer or producer the monopoly to either use specific industrial equipment or produce specific goods for a limited period. This monopoly, enforced by the appropriate government office, enabled an innovator to obtain a just reward for his efforts. In most countries the awarding of a patent prevents third parties from manufacturing and selling the product without the consent of the innovator. However, patents do encourage and protect the development of new ideas by the publication of new knowledge.

Originally each country issued its own patent laws, but by the mid-18th century it was recognized that patent rights should extend beyond national boundaries. The first international agreement was the **Paris Convention** of 1883. This has been revised on numerous occasions, the current treaties in operation being the Europeans Union's European Patent Convention (EPC) of 1978 and the Patent Cooperation Treaty (PCT) signed in Washington in 1970. The former is only open to European countries and administered by the European Patents Office (EPO). The latter is open to all countries of the world and is administered through the national patent offices of the country subscribing to the treaty.

The protection offered by a patent is of paramount importance to a company at the research, development and production stages of drug production. It is essential that a patent is filed as soon as new compounds have been made and shown to have interesting properties. Otherwise, a rival company working in the same field might pre-empt the patent, which means that a large amount of expensive research work would be unproductive in respect to company profits. In this respect, it is particularly important that the patent covers the relevant field and does not give a rival manufacturer an exploitable loophole.

The time required for the development of a drug from discovery to production can take at least 7–15 years. In many countries, patents normally run for 20 years from the date of application. Consequently, the time available for a manufacturer to recoup the cost of development and show a profit is rather limited, which accounts for the high cost of some new drugs. Furthermore, it also means that some compounds are never developed because the patent protected production time available to recoup the cost of development is too short.

11.8 Regulation

The release of a new drug onto the market must be approved by the regulating authority for that country. For example, in Britain this is the Medicines Control Agency (MCA), in the European Union it is the European Medicines Evaluation Agency (EMEA) and in the USA the US Food and Drugs Administration (FDA). These bodies, which are essentially consumer protection agencies, issue a so called **product licence** or **marketing authority (MA)** when they are satisfied as to the method of production, efficacy, safety and quality of the product. To obtain a product licence the pharmaceutical company is required to submit a comprehensive dossier that contains the relevant pharmacological, formulation and toxicological data and full details of all aspects of the production processes and dosage forms. The issuing of a product licence gives the pharmaceutical company or the person ordering its production the right, sometimes subject to conditions, to produce and sell the new product in the issuing country. Licences may be revoked if the producer does not strictly keep to the conditions laid down in the licence. Any changes, at a later date, to the production process, dosage forms or indications (usage) must also be approved and it is the responsibility of the company to carry out any additional tests that are required.

11.9 Questions

(1) (a) What is the critical path in drug development? (b) List the main stages in the critical path of the development of a drug.

(2) Explain the meaning of the terms (a) dosage form, (b) ELF, (c) telescoping in drug production, (d) excipient and (e) double blind trial.

(3) Outline the chemical factors that need to be considered when scaling up a research synthesis to pilot plant scale.

(4) Outline a possible production scale route for the preparation of the thromboxane analogue A.

(5) Explain the differences between (a) preclinical and clinical trials and (b) Phase I and Phase II trials.

(6) What is a patent? Why is it necessary to patent drugs?

Appendix

A.1   Sickle-cell anaemia

Sickle-cell anaemia is caused by a defective gene. This gene results in the replacement of the glutamate at position 6 of the β chains of haemoglobin (Hb) by a valine residue to produce sickle-cell haemoglobin (HbS). These HbS molecules aggregate into long polymer-like structures, which results in long sickle shaped red blood cells instead of the normal round cells. These red blood cells are able to transport oxygen in the normal fashion but their shape causes them to lodge in capillaries, which causes tissue damage and impairs blood circulation. This results in headaches, dizziness and ultimately death.

Fundamentals of Medicinal Chemistry, Edited by Gareth Thomas
© 2003 John Wiley & Sons, Ltd
ISBN 0 470 84306 3 (Hbk), ISBN 0 470 84307 1 (pbk)

A.2   Bacteria

Bacteria are microscopic plants varying in size from about 0.1 to 20 μ. They are usually unicellular and have a variety of shapes ranging from spheres to rods. Most bacteria have a well defined cell wall that covers the outer surface of the plasma membrane (see Appendix 3) of the cell. This is a rigid structure, consisting of a complex polypeptide–polysaccharide (peptidoglycan, Figures A2.2 and A2.3) matrix. It maintains the shape and integrity of the bacteria by preventing either the swelling and bursting (lysis) or the shrinking of the bacteria when the osmotic pressure of the surrounding medium changes. The bacterial cell wall is continually being broken down by enzymes in the surrounding medium and so it is continuously being rebuilt. This rebuilding process offers a potential target for drugs since inhibition of the reconstruction processes could destroy the integrity of the bacterial cell, resulting in its death.

Bacteria are commonly classified as being either Gram-positive or Gram-negative depending on their response to the Gram stain test. The cell walls of Gram-positive bacteria are about 25 nm thick and consist of up to 20 layers of the peptidoglycan (Figure A2.1(a)). In contrast, the cell walls of Gram-negative bacteria are only 2–3 nm thick and consist of an outer lipid bilayer attached through hydrophobic proteins and amide links to the peptidoglycan (Figure A2.1(b)). This lipid–peptidoglycan structure is separated from the plasma membrane by an aqueous compartment known as the **periplasmic space**. This space

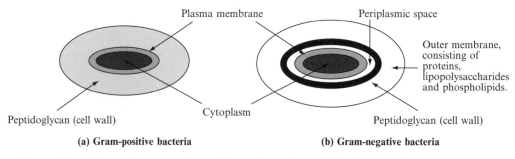

Figure A2.1   Schematic cross-sections of the cell envelopes of (a) Gram-positive and (b) Gram-negative bacteria

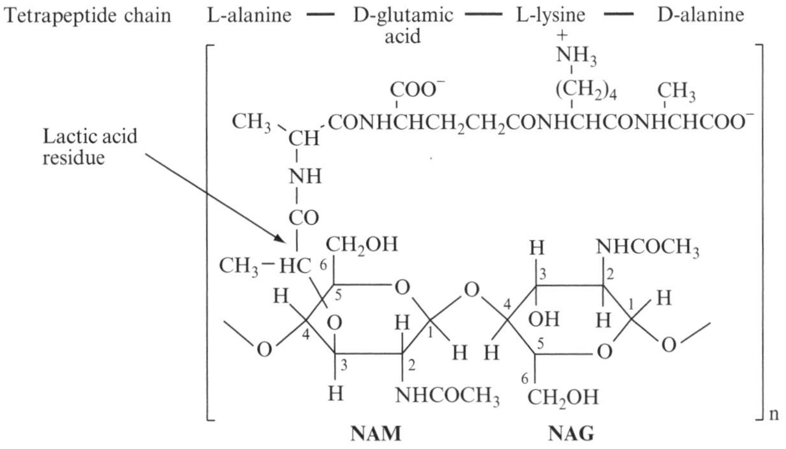

Figure A2.2   The structure of the monomer unit of the polyglycan of *S. aureus*. The cross links between chains are from the γ-amino group of the lysine to the carboxylate of the C-terminal D-alanine. The tetrapeptide can contain other amino acid residues

contains transport sugars, enzymes and other substances. The complete structure separating the cytoplasm of the bacteria from its surroundings is known as the **cell envelope**.

The peptidoglycans found in both Gram-positive and Gram-negative bacteria are commonly known as mureins. They are polymers composed of polysaccharide and peptide chains, which form a single, netlike molecule that completely surrounds the cell. The polysaccharide chains consist of alternating 1–4 linked β-N-acetylmuramic acid (NAM) and β-N-acetylglucosamine (NAG) units (Figure A2.2). Tetrapeptide chains are attached through the lactic acid residues of the NAM units of these polysaccharide chains.

In Gram-positive bacteria, the tetrapeptide chains of one polysaccharide chain are cross linked by pentaglycine peptide bridges from the γ-amino group of lysine to the terminal alanine of the tetrapeptide chains of a second polysaccharide chain to form a net-like polymer (Figure A2.3(a)). The pentaglycinepeptide bridges occasionally contain other residues. In Gram-negative bacteria the tetrapeptide chains are directly linked by amide group (peptide bond) bridges (Figure A2.3(b)). The structure is denser than that found in the Gram-positive cell wall because the peptidoglycan chains are closer together.

The exterior surface of Gram-positive bacteria is covered by **teichoic acids**. These are ribitol–phosphate or glycerol–phosphate polymer chains that are frequently substituted by alanine and glycosidically linked monosaccharides (Figure A2.4). They are attached to the peptidoglycan by a phosphate diester link. Teichoic acids can act as receptors to bacteriophages and some appear to have antigenic properties.

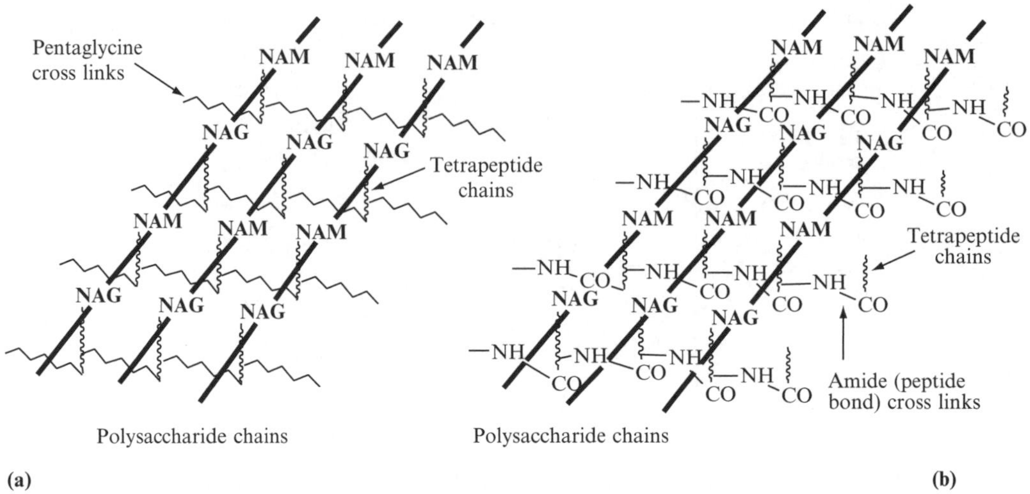

242   APPENDIX 2 BACTERIA

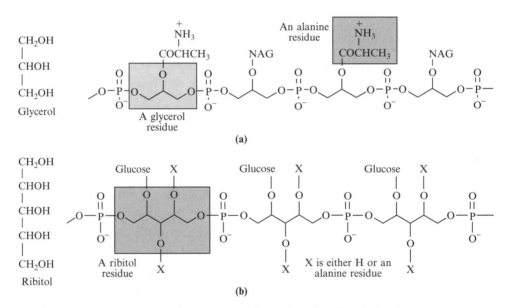

Figure A2.3 A schematic representation of the structure of the peptidoglycans of (a) Gram-positive and (b) Gram-negative bacteria

Figure A2.4 (a) A glycerol based teichoic acid. (b) A ribitol based teichoic acid. In many teichoic acids the monosaccharide residues are glucose and N-acetylglucosamine

The exterior surface of Gram-negative bacteria is more complex than that of the Gram-positive bacteria. It is coated with **lipopolysaccharides**, which largely consist of long chains of repeating oligosaccharide units that are attached to the outer membrane by a core oligosaccharide (Figure A2.5).

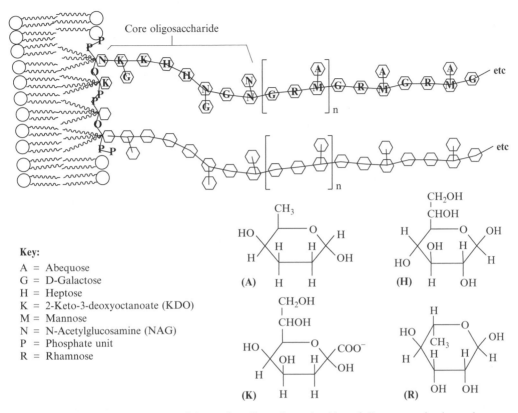

Key:

A = Abequose
G = D-Galactose
H = Heptose
K = 2-Keto-3-deoxyoctanoate (KDO)
M = Mannose
N = N-Acetylglucosamine (NAG)
P = Phosphate unit
R = Rhamnose

Figure A2.5 The structure of the surface lipopolysaccharides of Gram-negative bacteria

These lipopolysaccharides often contain monosaccharide units such as abequose (Abe) and 2-keto-3-deoxyoctanoate (KDO) that are rarely found in other organisms. The repeating units, which are known as **O-antigens**, are unique to a particular type of bacterium. Experimental evidence suggests that they play a part in the bacteria's recognition of host cells. It is also believed that they enable the host's immunological system to identify the invading bacteria and produce antibodies that destroy the bacteria. However, a particular bacterial cell can have a number of different O-antigens and it is this diversity that allows some bacteria to evade a host's immune system.

A.3   Cell membranes

Cells are broadly classified as either **prokaryotes** or **eukaryotes**. Prokaryotic cells are found in simpler organisms, such as bacteria. They do not have a membrane enclosed nucleus, but their DNA is dispersed in the cytoplasm of the cell. Eukaryotic cells are found in all members of the animal kingdom. Their structures contain distinct membrane encapsulated compartments, such as the nucleus, which contains their DNA, mitochondria and lysomes. These separate compartments are known as **organelles**.

All cells have a membrane, known as the **plasma** or **cytoplasmic membrane**, that separates the internal medium of a cell (**intracellular fluid**) from its surrounding medium (**extracellular fluid**). Membranes also form the boundaries between the various internal regions of the cell that retain the intracellular fluid in separate compartments in the cell. The plasma membrane maintains the integrity of the cell in its environment and also regulates the movement of substances into and out of the cell. These movements control health, as well as the flow of information between and within cells. The plasma membrane of a cell is also involved in both the generation and receipt of chemical and electrical signals, cell adhesion, which is responsible for tissue formation, cell locomotion, biochemical reactions and cell reproduction. The internal cell membranes have similar functions and, in addition, are often actively involved in the function of organelles. Most drugs have to pass through one or more membranes to reach their site of action.

The currently accepted structure of membranes (Figure A3.1) is a fluid-like bilayer arrangement of phospholipids with proteins and other substances such as steroids and glycolipids either associated with its surface or embedded in it to varying degrees. This structure is an intermediate state between the true liquid and solid states, with the lipid and protein molecules having a limited degree of rotational and lateral movement.

X-ray diffraction studies have shown that many naturally occurring membranes are about 5 nm thick. Experimental work has also shown that a potential difference exists across most membranes due to the movement of ions through pores in the membrane, known as **ion channels**, and the action of so called

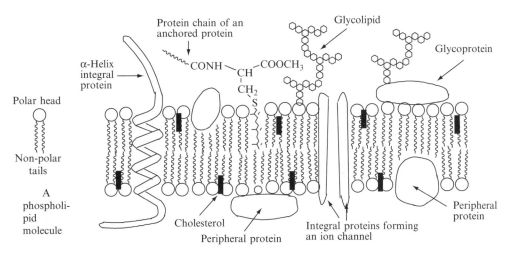

Figure A3.1 The fluid mosaic model of membranes. **Note:** Integral proteins either pass right through or are deeply embedded in the lipid bilayer. Peripheral proteins are attached to the surface of the lipid bilayer. Anchored proteins are attached to a so called anchor molecule embedded in the lipid bilayer.

chemical *pumps* in the membrane. The intracellular face of a membrane at rest, that is not undergoing cellular stimulation, is the negative side of the membrane. For a membrane at rest the potential difference (**resting potential**) between the two faces of the membrane varies from -20 to $-200\,mV$. However, when the membrane responds to cellular stimulation stimulation this inside face is depolarized and becomes positive.

A.4   Receptors

Receptors are specific areas of certain proteins and glycoproteins that are found either spanning cellular membranes or in the nuclei of living cells. Any endogenous or exogenous chemical agent that binds to a receptor is known as a **ligand**. The general region on a receptor where a ligand binds is known as the **binding domain**. It should be noted that the term **domain** is used to indicate any area of a bio-macromolecule that is linked to a specific function of that molecule. The binding of a drug to a receptor either inhibits or stimulates its action, which ultimately results in the physiological responses that are characteristic of the action of the drug. For example, some ligand–receptor interaction causes the opening or closing of ion channels, whist some interactions result in the release of so called **secondary messengers**, which promote a sequence of biochemical events that result in an appropriate physiological response (Figure A4.1). The mechanism by which the message carried by the ligand is translated through the receptor into a physiological response is known as **signal transduction**.

Receptors are classified according to function into four so called **superfamilies** of receptors (Table A4.1). The members of a superfamily will all have the same general structure and general mechanism of action. However, individual members of a superfamily tend to exhibit variations in the amino acid residue sequence in certain regions and also the sizes of their extracellular and intracellular domains. Each of these superfamilies is sub-divided into a number of types of receptor, whose members are usually defined by their endogenous ligand. For example, all receptors that bind acetylcholine (ACh) are of the cholinergic type and those that bind adrenaline and noradrenaline are of the adrenergic type. These sub-types are further classified either according to the type of genetic code responsible for their structure or after the exogenous ligands that selectively bind to the receptor. For example, the endogenous ligand acetylcholine will bind to all cholinergic receptors but the exogenic ligand nicotine will only bind to nicotinic

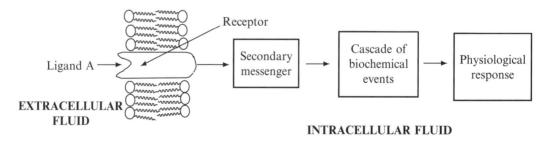

Figure A4.1   A schematic representation of signal transduction

Table A4.1   Superfamilies of receptors.

Superfamily	General notes concerning their action
Type 1	Opens ion channels.
Type 2	Binding causes a conformational change, which results in the attraction of a G-protein in the cytoplasm to an intracellular binding domain of the receptor molecule. This may either result in the opening or closing of an ion channel or the inhibition or activation of an enzyme.
Type 3	It is believed that the binding of a ligand to this type of receptor causes the receptor to dimerize. This is thought to result in conformational changes that cause the autophosphorylation of various tyrosine residues in the intracellular domain. These phosphorylated tyrosine sites act as high affinity binding sites for specific intercellular proteins.
Type 4	The members of this family occur in the nucleus of the cell. The N-terminal side of the receptor protein appears to control gene transcription.

cholinergic receptors (nAChR). Similarly muscarine will only bind to muscarinic cholinergic receptors (mAChR). However, it is possible to differentiate between different types of receptor within a sub-type. For example, three different types of muscarinic cholinergic receptor have been detected and a further two predicted from a study of the genes that code for this type of receptor. These five mAChR receptors are classified as m_n, where n is an integer form 1 to 5 inclusive.

Similar classifications are used for other receptors. For example, adrenoceptors are classified as α and β sub-types. These sub-types are further classified according to the nature of their exogenous ligands. The various types are distinguished by the use of subscript numbers.

The forces binding ligands to receptors covers the full spectrum of chemical bonding, namely covalent bonding, ionic bonding, dipole–dipole interactions of all types including hydrogen bonding, charge-transfer bonding, hydrophobic bonding and van der Waals' forces. The bonds between the ligand and the receptor are assumed to be formed spontaneously when the ligand reaches the appropriate distance from its receptor for bond formation.

The binding of many drugs to their receptors is by weak reversible interactions.

$$\text{drug} + \text{receptor} \rightleftharpoons \text{drug} - \text{receptor} \qquad (A4.1)$$

This means that the binding of a drug to its receptor is concentration dependent.

As the concentration of the ligand in the extracellular fluid increases, equilibrium (A4.1) will move to the right and the drug will bind to the receptor.

However, when the concentration of the drug in the extracellular fluid falls, the equilibrium will move to the left and the drug–receptor complex will dissociate. Consequently, drugs and endogenous ligands become ineffective as soon as their concentrations fall below a certain limit as an insufficient number of receptors are being activated by these ligands. Endogenous reduction of drug concentration is brought about by metabolism and excretion. Consequently, both these processes will have a direct bearing on the duration of action of a drug.

Drugs that form strong bonds with their receptors do not readily dissociate from the receptor when their concentrations in the extracellular fluid fall. Consequently, drugs that act in this manner will often have a long duration of action. This is a useful attribute for drugs used in the treatment of cancers, where it is particularly desirable that the drug forms irreversible bonds to the receptors of tumour cells.

A.5 Transfer through membranes

Substances are transported through membranes by osmosis, filtration, passive diffusion, facilitated diffusion, active transport, endocytosis and exocytosis. **Passive diffusion** is the major route for the transport of drugs across membranes. It occurs down a concentration gradient from a high to a low concentration. In passive diffusion the drug dissolves into the lipid membrane from the aqueous medium, diffuses across the membrane and dissolves out of the membrane into the aqueous medium. Since the interiors of membranes are nonpolar, passive diffusion is most effective for uncharged nonpolar species. Charged and highly polar species are not easily transported through a membrane by passive diffusion. However, a potential drug must have sufficient polar character to penetrate the hydrophilic surface of the membrane. Consequently, the structures of potential drugs must contain a balanced ratio of lipid solubilizing regions to water solubilizing regions if a sufficient concentration of the compound is to cross a membrane by passive diffusion.

Active transport is also an important route for the transfer of drugs through a membrane by a so called **carrier protein**. The solute combines with a specific protein in the membrane, causing this protein to change its conformation. This change results in the transport of the solute from one side of the membrane to the other, where it is released into the aqueous medium. The rate of active transport is dependent on the concentration of the solute at the absorption sites. It follows first order kinetics at concentrations less than those required to saturate the available carriers but changes to zero order at concentrations above the saturation point. Consequently, increasing a drug's concentration above the saturation limit in the extracellular fluid does not increase the rate at which the drug is delivered to its active site. Active transport usually operates from a low concentration to a high concentration, which requires the cell to expend large quantities of energy.

Carrier proteins are highly selective, transporting solutes with specific chemical structures. As they are normally involved in the transport of many naturally occurring compounds they will often transport drugs with structures related to these natural products. This type of structural relationship can be use in the approach to the design of new drugs.

Facilated diffusion also involves the use of a carrier protein. It differs from active transport in that it occurs from a high to a low concentration and so does not require energy to be supplied by the cell. However, falicilated diffusion appears to play a minor role in the transport of drugs through membranes.

A.6   Regression analysis

In medicinal chemistry, it is often desirable to obtain mathematical relationships in the form of equations between sets of data, which have been obtained from experimental work or calculated using theoretical considerations. Regression analysis is a group of mathematical methods used to obtain such relationships. The data is fed into a suitable computer program, which on execution produces an equation that represents the line that is the best fit for that data. For example, an investigation indicated that the relationship between the activity and the partition coefficients of a number of related compounds appeared to be linear (Figure A6.1). Consequently, this data could be represented mathematically in the form of the straight line equation $y = mx + c$. Regression analysis would calculate the values of m and c that gave the line of best fit to the data. When one is dealing with a linear relationship the analysis is usually carried out using the method of least squares.

Regression equations do not indicate the accuracy and spread of the data. Consequently, they are normally accompanied by additional data, which as a minimum requirement should include the number of observations used (n), the standard deviation of the observations (s) and the correlation coefficient (r).

The value of the correlation coefficient is a measure of how closely the data matches the equation. It varies from zero to one. A value of $r = 1$ indicates a perfect match. In medicinal chemistry r values greater than 0.9 are usually regarded as representing an acceptable degree of accuracy, provided they are obtained using a reasonable number of results with a suitable standard deviation.

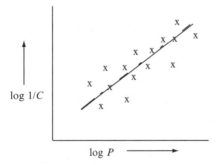

Figure A6.1   A hypothetical plot of the activity (log1/C) of a series of compounds against the logarithm of their partition coefficients (log P)

The value of $100r^2$ is a measure of the percentage of the data that can satisfactorily explained by the regression analysis. For example, a value of $r = 0.90$ indicates that 81 per cent of the results can be satisfactorily explained by regression analysis using the parameters specified. It indicates that 19 per cent of the data is not satisfactorily explained by these parameters and so indicates that the use of an additional parameter(s) might give a more acceptable account of the results. Suppose, for example, regression analysis using an extra parameter gave a regression constant of 0.98. This shows that 96.04 per cent of the data is now satisfactorily accounted for by the chosen parameters.

A.7   Enzymes

Enzymes are large protein molecules (**apoenzymes**), which act as catalysts for almost all the chemical reactions that occur in living organisms. The structures of a number of enzymes contains groups of metal ions, known as metal **clusters**, coordinated to the peptide chain. These enzymes are often referred to as **metalloenzymes**. Many enzymes require the presence of organic compounds (**co-enzymes**) and/or metal ions and inorganic compounds (**co-factors**) in order to function. These composite active enzyme systems are known as **holoenzymes**.

apoenzyme + co-enzyme and/or co-factor = holoenzyme

(*inactive*)   (*inactive*)   (*active*)

Enzymes are found embedded in cell walls and membranes as well as occuring in the various fluids found in living organisms. A number of enzymes are produced in specific areas of the body by the metabolism of inactive protein precursors known as **proenzymes** or **zymogens**.

proenzyme $\rightleftharpoons$ active form of the enzyme

This allows the body to produce the active form of the enzyme only in the region of the body where it is required.

Enzymes are broadly classified into six major types (Table A7.1). Those that catalyse the same reactions but have significantly different structures are known as **isofunctional** enzymes.

The International Union of Biochemistry has recommended that enzymes have three names, namely a systematic name, which shows the reaction being catalysed and the type of reaction based on the classification in Table A7.1, a recommended trivial name and a four figure Enzyme Commission code (EC code). Nearly all systematic and trivial enzyme names have the suffix **-ase**. Systematic names show, often in semi-chemical equation form, the conversion the enzyme promotes and the class of the enzyme. Trivial names are usually based on the function of the enzyme but may also include or be based on the name of the substrate. However, some trivial names in current use are historical and bear no relationship to the action of the enzyme or its substrate, for example, pepsin and trypsin are the names commonly used for two enzymes that catalyse the breakdown of proteins during digestion. The Enzyme Commission's code is unique for each enzyme. It is based on the classification in Table A7.1 but further subdivides each class of enzyme according to how it functions. The full code is

Table A7.1   The classification of enzymes

Code	Classification	Type of reaction catalysed
1	Oxidoreductases	Oxidations and reductions
2	Transferases	The transfer of a group from one molecule to another
3	Hydrolases	Hydrolysis of various functional groups
4	Lyases	Cleavage of a bond by nonoxidative and nonhydrolytic mechanisms
5	Isomerases	The interconversion of all types of isomer
6	Ligases (synthases)	The formation of a bond between molecules

given in the International Union of Biochemistry (IUB) publication **Enzyme Nomenclature**. This text uses trivial names, as they are usually easier to read in print. In addition, some letter abbreviations are also used.

In its simplest form, the catalytic action of enzymes is believed to depend on the substrate or substrates, binding to the surface of the enzyme. This binding usually occurs on a specific part of the enzyme known as its **active site**. Once the substrate (S) or substrates are bound to the surface of the enzyme (E) reaction takes place and the products (P) are formed and released, whilst the enzyme is recycled into the system.

$$E + S \rightleftharpoons E\text{–}S \text{ complex} \rightleftharpoons E\text{–}P \text{ complex} \rightleftharpoons P + E$$
$$\text{Recycled}$$

It is believed that an enzyme considerably reduces the activation energy required for each of the stages in an enzyme controlled reaction (Figure A7.1).

Active sites are usually visualized as either pockets, clefts or indentations in the surface of the enzyme. The amino acid residues forming the site can be located some distance apart in the peptide chain but are brought together by the folding of the peptide chain. The binding of a substrate to an active site is believed to involve a mutual change in the conformations of both the substrate and the enzyme. These changes allow the substrate to bind in the exact position necessary for reaction, which explains why enzymes are more effective than chemical catalysts in increasing the rates of reaction. The change in conformation caused by a substrate binding to the active site can also result in the formation of another active site, known as an **allosteric site**, on the enzyme. This behaviour is known as **allosteric activation**. It occurs with increasing concentration of the substrate and increases the capacity of the enzyme to process substrate.

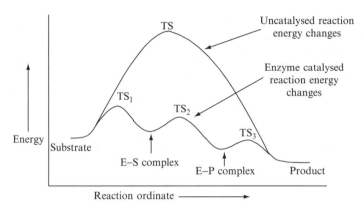

Figure A7.1 The effect of an enzyme on the minimum energy pathway of a simple enzyme catalysed reaction involving a single substrate. (TS = transition state.) The heights of the energy barriers TS$_1$, TS$_2$ and TS$_3$ will vary depending on which step in the enzyme controlled route is the rate controlling step

   The chemical activity of a cell must be controlled in order for the cell to function correctly. Enzymes offer a means of controlling that activity in that they can be switched from active to inactive states by changes induced in their conformations. Compounds that modulate the action of enzymes and other molecules by these conformational changes are known as **regulators**, **modulators** or **effectors**. These compounds may switch on (activators) or switch off (inhibitors) an enzyme. They may be generally classified for convenience as either compounds that covalently modify the enzyme or allosteric regulators. The former type of regulation involves the attachment of a chemical group to the enzyme by covalent bonding, which may either inactivate or activate an enzyme.
   Allosteric control involves the reversible binding of a compound to an allosteric site referred to as a **regulatory site** on the enzyme. These compounds may be either one of the compounds involved in the metabolic pathway (**feedback regulators**) or a compound that is not a product of the metabolic pathway. In both cases, the binding usually results in conformational changes, which either activate or deactivate the enzyme. Proenzymes also act as a form of enzyme control.

A.8   Prostaglandins

The prostaglandins are a group of naturally occurring compounds whose molecular structures are based on that of prostanoic acid.

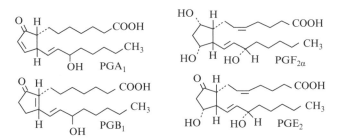

Prostaglandins are associated with the pathology of inflammation and fever. They were believed to be synthesized in the prostate gland (hence the name) but are now known to be synthesized throughout the body. A number of different prostaglandins have been isolated and identified. They may be named using the IUPAC system but are more commonly referred to by a series of abbreviations that use PG to indicate a prostaglandin. These abbreviations are based on the classification of the prostaglandins into families. The members of a family differ only in the number, position and configuration of the alkene $C = C$ bonds in the side chains and are distinguished by the use of a capital letter after PG (Figure A8.1). Numerical subscripts following the final letter indicate the number and configuration of the alkene double bonds that occur in the chains attached to the five membered ring. An exception to this rule are the subscripts α and β, which are used to distinguish between the sub-groups of the PGF family based on its 9α and 9β isomers respectively.

Figure A8.1   Examples of the structures and abbreviations used for prostaglandins

A.9 Cancer

Cancer is a disease that can occur in all types of body tissue. It is found in many forms, including solid tissue formations (tumours or neoplasms), leukaemias (blood cancer) and lymphomas (cancer of the lymphoid cells). Cancers are due to a reduction in control or loss of control of the growth of cells. This leads to a proliferation of cell growth. In its early stages the cells formed by this growth resemble the parent but as the cancer progresses they lose the appearance and function of the parent cell. This loss of function if left unchecked will become life threatening. For example, a growing tumour will obstruct, block and generally affect adjacent organs. If these are nerves it will cause pain. Furthermore, cancer cells are invasive. As the cancer grows, the cells lose their adhesion and the malignant cells are carried in the blood to other parts of the body. These cells lodge in different parts of the body and grow into so called secondary cancers.

A.10 Viruses

Viruses are not classified as living organisms since they require the use of the host cell's biological system in order to reproduce. They are infective agents that are smaller than bacteria. Viruses are essentially packages of chemicals, known as **virons**, that are able to penetrate a host cell's membrane. However, a particular virus is only able to invade specific types of host cells. Once inside the host cell the virus uses the hosts cell's biological systems to form multiple copies of its own proteins and nucleic acids. These new proteins and nucleic acids may directly cause a pathological condition and/or may be assembled into new virons in the host cell. The new virons are released from the host by either lysis or a biological process called budding. The former causes the death of the cell, whilst the latter does not always result in the death of the host cell. However, in both cases, the virons are liberated into the extracellular fluid and are now able to infect other host cells.

Viruses contain a central core of either RNA or DNA fully or partially surrounded by a protein coating called a **capsid** (Figure A10.1(a)). **Capsomers** are the individual proteins that form the capsid. Enveloped viruses have an additional external lipoprotein envelope that surrounds the capsid (Figure A10.1(b)). Viruses are broadly divided into **RNA viruses, RNA retroviruses** and **DNA viruses** according to their mode of action and structure. In RNA viruses, viral RNA replication occurs almost entirely in the cytoplasm. The viral mRNA used to produce viral proteins either forms part of the RNA carried by the virus or is synthesized by an enzyme already present in the viron. However, RNA retroviruses synthesize viral DNA using their RNA as a template and viral enzyme systems known as **reverse transcriptases**. This viral DNA is incorporated into the host genome to form a so called **provirus**. Transcription of the provirus forms viral mRNA, which is used to produce viral proteins. Most DNA viruses form viral mRNA by transcription of the viral DNA using the host cell's polymerases. Some of the viral proteins produced using this viral mRNA are enzymes that catalyse the production of more viral DNA. Antiviral drugs act by either inhibiting viral nucleic acid synthesis, inhibiting attachment to and penetration of the host cell or inhibiting viral protein synthesis.

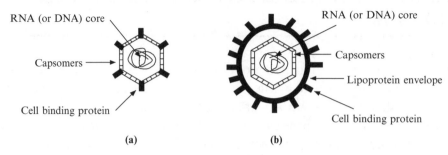

Figure A10.1 A schematic representation of the structure of a virus (a) without a lipoprotein envelope and (b) with a lipoprotein envelope

A.11 Blood–brain barrier

The blood vessels that carry substances around the body are lined with so called endothelial tissue made up of so called endothelial cells. The gaps between these endothelial cells that form the endothelial tissue varies depending on the function of the blood vesel. For example, in the kidney the gaps are comparatively large, thereby allowing relatively large chemical species to diffuse through the tissue. However, the single layer of endothelial cells that line the capillaries of the brain forms a structure that is known as the **blood–brain barrier**, in which the gaps between the endothelial cells are extremely small. This means that nearly all the substances entering the brain have to pass through the endothelial cell membranes, that is, through the blood–brain barrier. This makes it more difficult for polar substances to enter the brain unless they are actively transported (see Appendix 5). Consequently, this factor must be taken into account when designing drugs to target the brain. Another factor is the fact that the blood–brain barrier also contains enzymes that protect the brain.

A.12   Enzyme structure and species

The structure of a specific enzyme may vary from species to species. These differences, which tend to be the replacement of one or a few amino acid residue by alternative residues, may be important in that they may form selective targets for drugs. For example, differences in the structures of human and bacterial DHFR result in the antibacterial trimethoprin binding specifically to bacterial DHFR (see section 7.5.1).

The structure of an enzyme can also vary within a person, since different genes may encode enzymes that catalyse the same reaction. These enzymes are known as **isozymes**. Isozymes are often specific for different types of tissue. For example, lactate dehydrogenase (LDH) is produced in two forms, the M-type (muscle) and the H-type (heart). The M-type is predominates in tissue subject to anaerobic conditions, such as skeletal muscle and liver tissue, whereas the H-type predominates in tissue under aerobic conditions, such as the heart. Isozymes may be used as a diagnostic aid. For example, the presence of H-type LDH in the blood indicates a heart attack, since heart attacks cause the death of heart muscle with the subsequent release of H-type LDH into the circulatory system.

Variations in the structures of enzymes within a species can also occur between and within ethnic groups of the same species. For example, a number of different alcohol dehydrogenase isoenzymes have been observed in some Asians.

Answers to questions

Numerical answers may be slightly different from the ones you obtain due to differences in calculating methods and equipment. However, a correct answer is one that approximates to the given answer. Answers that require the writing of notes are answered by either an outline of the points that should be included in the answer or a reference to the appropriate section(s) of the text. Where questions have more than one correct answer only one answer is given.

Chapter 1

(1) See the appropriate figure or table: (a) Figure 1.1, (b) Figure 1.28(a), (c) Table 1.5, (d) Figure 1.1, (e) Figure 1.5(a) and (f) Figure 1.22.

(2) (a) A nonpeptide residue incorporated as an integral part of a protein.
　　(b) The amide group linking the amino acid residues together in peptides and proteins.
　　(c) The disulphide bonds that cross link two peptide chains in a protein.
　　(d) The overall shape of a protein molecule.

(3) (a) See Section 1.4, (b) see section 1.4.1, (c) see section 1.4.1, (d) see section 1.4.1, (e) see Figure 1.12.

(4) Select five from fatty acids, acylglycerols, steroids, terpenes, phospholipids and glycolipids. (a) See Table 1.5. (b) See Table 1.7.

(5) See Section 1.5.4. The saturated six membered rings are normally in a chair conformation whilst the saturated five membered rings have an envelope conformation.

(6) (a) See Section 1.6. (b) See section 1.6.3. (c) See section 1.6.5.

(7) (a) TTAGGCATCG, (b) AAUGGCUACG.

Fundamentals of Medicinal Chemistry, Edited by Gareth Thomas
© 2003 John Wiley & Sons, Ltd
ISBN 0 470 84306 3 (Hbk), ISBN 0 470 84307 1 (pbk)

(8) (a) The main differences are the following.

- DNA molecules usually have a very large RMM value compared to RNA molecules.
- The structure of RNA contains the sugar residue ribose whilst that of DNA contains the sugar deoxyribose.
- RNA molecules consist of a single strand of nucleotides whilst DNA molecules consist of two nucleotide strands in the form of a supercoiled double helix.

  (b) See Section 1.6.5.

(9) The first four codons are not involved in protein synthesis. Protein synthesis starts with AUG and stops with UAA. The peptide coded by the codons between the stop and start signals is

Met–Pro–Arg–Gly–Gly–Try

Chapter 2

(1) (a) See Section 2.3. (b) See section 2.6. (c) See section 2.6. (d) See section 2.3. (e) See section 2.7.1.

(2) The nature of the pathological target. Its site of action, the nature of the desired action, its stability, ease of absorption and distribution, metabolism, dosage form and regimen.

(3) See Section 2.6.

(4) For definitions see Section 2.7. The factors affecting the pharmacokinetic phase are ADME. The factor affecting the pharmacodynamic phase is the stereoelectronic structure of the drug molecule.

(5) The reduction in pH reduces the negative charge of the albumin and so increases its electrophilic character. Therefore, as amphetamine molecules are nucleophilic in nature, their binding should improve with decrease in pH. Part of this binding will will involve salt formation between the amphetamine and the albumin. Amphetamine is more likely to form salts in which it acts as the positive ion as the electrophilic nature of the albumin decreases with increase in pH.

(6) See Table 2.1.

Chapter 3

(1) See Section 3.1.

(2) See Section 3.2.1. (i) Replacing a rigid structure by an equivalent sized rigid structure gives a better chance of an active analogue. The shape of a rigid structure may give information about the size and shape of its receptor provided the rigid part of the molecule is the part that binds to the receptor. If the part of a ligand that binds to the receptor is a rigid structure it can also indicate the best conformation for analogues to bind to the receptor.
(ii) Different conformations can result in different activities and potencies.
(iii) See section 3.2.3 and Table 2.1.

(3) Compounds that are reasonably water soluble are more easily absorbed, transported to their site of action and eliminated from the body.

(4) (i) High polar group to carbon atom ratio (see section 3.4).
(ii) The presence of polar groups that can hydrogen bond to water molecules and ionize in water (see section 3.4 and Figure 3.5).

(5) (i) Form salts that would improve water solubility but would break down to yield the drug in the biological system (see section 3.5).
(ii) Introduce water solubilizing groups into a part of the structure that is not the pharmacophore of the drug (see section 3.6).
(iii) The use of special dosage forms (see section 3.4).

(6) See Figure 3.6. for methods
(i) O-acylation with succinic anhydride.
(ii) O- or N-alkylation with an appropriate reagent.

Chapter 4

(1) Structure–activity relationship. SARs are the general relationships obtained from a study of the changes in activity with changes in the structure of a lead. These changes are used to find or predict the structure with the optimum activity. For example, see Figure 4.1.

(2) (i) See Table 4.2. (ii) CF_3. It is approximately the same size as a chlorine atom.

(3) See Section 4.3.2 and Table 4.3 for both parts (i) and (ii).

(4) See Table 4.2 for all the answers to parts (i)–(iii).

(5) See Section 4.4.

(6) Lipophilicity: see section 4.4.1 (P and π). Shape: see section 4.4.3 (E_s and MR). Electronic effects: see section 4.4.2 (σ).

(7) (a) See Section 4.4.4.
    (b) (i) $n =$ the number of compounds used to derive the equation; $s =$ the standard deviation for the equation; $r =$ the regression constant, the nearer its value to units the better the fit of the data to the Hansch equation. Equations are normally said to have an acceptable degree of accuracy if r is greater than 0.9.
      (ii) See Section 4.4.4 and in particular Equation (4.11).
      (iii) A more polar substituent would have a negative π value (see Table 4.4), which could reduce the activity of the compound.

(8) (a) See Section 4.4.4.1
    (b) Substituents in the upper right hand corner of Figure 4.6.

(9) (i) See Section 4.5.
   (ii) Can only be used for substituents listed in the two decision trees.
     The lead compound must have an unfused aromatic ring.
     It requires a rapid method of assessing the biological activity of the lead and its analogues.

Chapter 5

(1) See Figure 5.1(b), Figure 5.3(a) and Figure 5.3(c).

(2) (a) See Section 5.2. (b) See Equation (5.1) in section 5.2.

$$\text{(c)} \quad E_{\text{coulombic}} = \frac{Q_{C_1} Q_{C_2}}{Dr_{C_{1-2}}} + \frac{(Q_{C_1} Q_{C_H})}{Dr_{C_1 - H}} + 3\frac{(Q_{C_2} Q_{C_H})}{Dr_{C_2 - H}}$$

where Q represents the point charge on the specified atoms and r the distance between the specified atoms.

(d) **Advantages:** less computing time, very large molecules may be modelled and can be used to give information on the binding of ligands to the target site. **Disadvantages:** accuracy of the structure depends on selecting the correct force field and parameter values. Structures are normally determined at zero Kelvin so they will have different conformations at room and body temperatures.

(3) See Section 5.2.1 and Figure 5.5. Link the fragments methanoic acid and methane to form the acetyl side chain. Link this side chain and methanoic acid to benzene. Check the hybridization of the atom is correct and energy minimize.

(4) See Section 5.2.1 and in particular Figure 5.6.

(5) (a) See Figure 5.3. (b) See section 5.5.

(6) (a) It is based on the concept that all material particles exhibit wavelike properties. This means that the mathematics of wave mechanics can be used to describe and predict these properties.
(b) **Schrodinger equation:** $H\Psi = E\Psi$

(c) **Advantages:** useful for calculating the values of physical properties of structure, the electron distribution in a structure and the most likely points at which a molecule will react with electrophiles and nucleophiles. **Disadvantages:** can only be used for structures that contain several hundred atoms. Requires a great deal of computing time.

Chapter 6

(1) See Sections 6.1 and 6.1.1.

(2) The objectives of the synthesis; do they require the formation of a library of separate compounds or mixtures?
The size of the library.
Solid or solution phase.
If solid phase is selected, use parallel synthesis or Furka's mix and split?
The nature of the building blocks and their ease of availability.
The suitability of the reactions in the sequence.
The method of identification of the structure of the final products.
The nature of the screening tests and procedures.

(3) See Sections 6.2.1 and 6.2.2.

(4) See Section 6.2.2. Adapt the scheme given in Figure 6.9. Use one of the encoding methods described in section 6.3.

(5) See Section 6.3.

(6) See Section 6.5.

Chapter 7

(1) (a) See Section 7.2.1. (b) See Section 7.4. (c) See Section 7.2.

(2) See section 7.2.2 for definitions and mode of action. When the concentrations of the ions being transferred by the ionophore are the same on both sides of the membrane.

(3) See Section 7.2.2. By inactivation of the drug by hydrolysis of the β-lactam ring.

(4) See Section 7.3.1 and 7.3.2.

(5) See Section 7.3.2. The drug candidate must bind to the enzyme's active site and must contain a group that is converted by the enzyme to a group that can react with the enzyme's active site.

(6) See Section 7.3.3.

(7) See Section 7.4.2.

(8) See Section 7.5.1.

(9) See Section 7.5.4. They form either interstrand or intrastrand links, which prevents DNA replication.

(10) See Section 7.5.5.

(11) See Section 7.6.

Chapter 8

(1) See Sections (a) 8.2, (b) 8.4.1, (c) 8.4.2, (d) 8.5.

(2) Absolute bioavailability (Equation (8.28)) and half-life (Equation (8.5)) as a measure of the rate of elimination. These parameters would give an indication of the relative effectiveness of each of the compounds. Absolute bioavailability would indicate the compound with the best absorption characteristics, whilst half-life would show which compound was the most stable *in situ* and so would have the best chance of being therapeutically effective.

(3) Plot a graph of log C against t. The slope is equal to $k_{el}/2.303$. (i) $1.84\,h^{-1}$, (ii) $4.12\,dm^3$, (iii) $7.58\,dm^3\,h^{-1}$. The assumption made is that the elimination exhibits first order kinetics.

(4) At one minute, if the clearance rate is $5\,cm^3\,min^{-1}$, $5\,cm^3$ will be clear of the drug, that is, 5/50 of the drug will have been removed, leaving 45 mg of the drug in the compartment. In the next minute another 5/50th of the remaining amount of the drug will be removed, as the clearance rate is constant, but this will be removed from the 45 mg, leaving 40.5 mg, and so on. The figures corresponding to the times are

Time lapse (minutes):   1   2   3   4   5   6   7   8   9   10
Drug remaining (mg): 45 40.5 36.5 32.8 29.5 26.5 23.8 21.4 19.3 17.4

A logarithmic plot using logarithms to **base 10** of the concentration against time is a straight line with a slope of 0.4584. Assuming a first order elimination process, the value of k_{el} (see Figure 8.6) calculated from this slope is

$$2.303 \times 0.4584 = 1.056$$

and the value of $t_{1/2}$ calculated from k_{el} using Equation (8.5) is 0.0656 minutes.

(5) Absolute bioavailability is defined by Equation (8.28); the values of the IV data required are the answers to question (3).

 (1) Calculate the AUC for the intravenously administered dose by substituting Equation (8.10) in Equation (8.12). This gives

$$\text{AUC for the IV} = \frac{\text{administered dose}}{V_d k_{el}} = \frac{30}{4.12 \times 1.84} = 3.96$$

(2) Substitute this value in Equation (8.28) to give the absolute bioavailability:

$$\text{absolute bioavailability} = \frac{5.01/50}{3.96/30} = 0.76$$

This value indicates that the IV bolus administration gives a significantly better bioavailability than oral administration.

(6) The parameters that could be used to compare the biological activities of the analogues are the following.

Half-life (calculate using Equation (8.5)), which would give a measure of the duration of the action. The longer the half-life the longer the time the drug is available in the body.

Absolute bioavailability (calculate using Equation (8.28)). The bigger the absolute bioavailability the greater the chance of a favourable biological action.

Analogue:	A	B	C	D
Half-life (minutes):	5	25	15	40
Absolute bioavailability:	1.036	1.526	0.812	1.175

The best analogue is D because it has the longest half-life and a reasonable bioavailability.

(7) $C_{ss} = k_0/Cl_p$ and $Cl_p = V_d k_{el}$

Calculate k_{el} from the value of $t_{1/2}$ (use Equation (8.5)).

$$t_{1/2} = 0.2772\,h^{-1}$$

Convert V_d to cm^3 and calculate the value of Cl_p. Substitute Cl_p in the expression for C_{ss}. Answer: rate of infusion $= 4.35\,\mu g\,cm^3\,h^{-1}$.

Chapter 9

(1) (a) See Section 9.1. (b) See Section 9.8.1 and 9.8.2.

(2) See Section 9.1.2. and 9.1.4.

(3) See Section 9.2, especially Table 9.1.

(4) See Table 9.3. The amide bond and the carboxylic acid group make the conjugate more water soluble than the original aromatic acid.

(5) (a)

Hydroxylation of the benzene ring.

$COOC_2H_5$

Hydrolysis of the ester to

CH_3

Cleavage of the N-CH$_3$ bond to

$COOH$ + C_2H_5OH

CH_3

$HCHO$ + Ph $COOC_2H_5$ (N–H)

(b) Hydroxylation of the benzene ring.

—N=N—⟨⟩—NH$_2$ ⟶ ⟨⟩—N=N—⟨⟩—NHCOCH$_3$

Acylation

Reductive cleavage

⟨⟩—NH$_2$ H$_2$N—⟨⟩—NH$_2$

(6) (a) To inactive the drug. Metabolism to inert metabolites that are sufficiently water soluble to be readily excreted via the kidney.

(b) The α-carbon of an ethyl group t-amine is hydroxylated and cleaved to form methanal and the N-methylaminobenzene. Methanal could be excreted via the lungs or be metabolized further to ethanoic acid. The N-methylaminobenzene could be metabolically oxidized to the corresponding N-hydroxy compound or dealkylated to aminobenzene and methanal.

(7) (a) A is metabolized faster than the drug, so it does not accumulate in the body.
(b) B to C is the main metabolic route, since this is a very much faster process than B to F.
(c) C to D; C will accumulate in the body. If C is pharmacologically active this could pose potential clinical problems for a patient.

(8) To avoid fatal over-doses.

(9) See Section 9.8.3. Use a N-methyldihydropyridine derivative as carrier. This carrier would require a substituent group that can bond to the dopamine diethanoate. The best group for this purpose is probably a carboxylic acid group, since amides are slowly hydrolysed. This means the prodrug has a good chance of reaching the blood–brain barrier in sufficient quantity to be effective. Once the prodrug has

entered the brain, it is easily oxidized to the quaternary salt, which because of its charge cannot return across the blood–brain barrier.

Chapter 10

(1) (i), (ii) See Section 10.2. (iii) See section 10.1.

(2) See Section 10.2.

(3) See Section 10.2.3.

(4) See Figure 10.10. Use propyliodide instead of ethyliodide in Figure 10.10.

(5) Synthon, see Section 10.3.1.

(i)

(ii)

(iii) A pericyclic disconnection.

(iv) A pericyclic disconnection.

(6) FGI, see section 10.3.1.

(i)

(ii)

Chapter 11

(1) (a) See Section 11.1. (b) List is the activities given in Figure 11.1.

(2) (a) See Section 11.5. (b) See section 11.2.2 and Equation (11.1) for a definition. (c) See Section 11.2.3. (d) See section 11.5. (e) See section 11.3.

(3) See Section 11.2 and 11.4.

(4) Use the route given in Figure 11.5. Use dimethoxypropane to form the dioxan ring (see the corresponding stage in Figure 11.4).

(5) (a) See Section 11.3. (b) See Section 11.3.

(6) See Section 11.7.

Selected further reading

Drug safety

Glaxo Group Research, *Drug Safety, a Shared Responsibility*, Churchill Livingstone, 1991.

General chemistry

G. Thomas, *Chemistry for Pharmacy and the Life Sciences including Pharmacology and Biomedical Science*, Prentice-Hall, 1996.
J. G. Morris, *A Biologists Physical Chemistry*, Second Edition, Arnold, 1974.

Synthetic chemistry

S. Warren, *Organic Synthesis, the Disconnection Approach*, Wiley, 1982.
R. S. Ward, *Selectivity in Organic Synthesis*, Wiley, 1999.
A. N. Collins, G. N. Sheldrake and J. Crosby (Editors), *Chiralty in Industry. The Commercial Manufacture and Applications of Optically Active Compounds*, Wiley, 1992.

Biochemistry

T. M. Devlin, (Ed), *Textbook of Biochemistry with Clinical Correlations*, Fourth Edition, Wiley–Liss, 1997.
D. Voet, J. G. Voet and C. W. Pratt, *Fundamentals of Biochemistry*, Wiley, 1999.

Pharmacology

H. P. Rang, M. M. Dale and J. M. Ritter, *Pharmacology*, Third Edition, Churchill Livingstone, 1995.

Fundamentals of Medicinal Chemistry, Edited by Gareth Thomas
© 2003 John Wiley & Sons, Ltd
ISBN 0 470 84306 3 (Hbk), ISBN 0 470 84307 1 (pbk)

Inorganic medicinal chemistry

S. J. Lippard and J. M. Berg, *Principles of Bioinorganic Chemistry*, University Science, 1994.

Medicinal chemistry

J. N. Delgado and W. A. Remers (Eds), *Wilson and Gisvold's Textbook of Organic Medicinal and Pharmaceutical Chemistry*, 10th Edition, Lippincott-Raven, 1998.

G. Thomas, *Medicinal Chemistry, an Introduction*, Wiley, 2000.

H. J. Smith (Ed), *Smith and Williams' Introduction to the Principles of Drug Design and Action*, Third Edition, Harwood, 1998.

T. Nogrady, *Medicinal Chemistry*, Second Edition, Oxford University Press, 1988.

M. E. Wolf (Ed), *Burgers Medicinal Chemistry*, Fifth Edition, Wiley, 1997.

D. Lednicer (Ed), *Chronicles of Drug Discovery*, various volumes, Wiley, various dates.

Combinatorial chemistry

S. R. Wilson and A. W. Czarnick (Eds), *Combinatorial Chemistry, Synthesis and Application*, Wiley, 1997.

N. K. Terrett, *Combinatorial Chemistry*, Oxford University Press, 1998.

Metabolism

G. Gibson and P. Skett, *Introduction to Drug Metabolism*, Third Edition, Nelson Thornes, 2001.

Pharmaceutics

M. Rowland and T. N. Tozer, *Clinical Pharmacokinetics*, Third Edition, Williams and Wilkins, 1995.

A. T. Florence and P. Atwood, *Physicochemical Principles of Pharmacy*, Third Edition, Macmillan, 1998.

A. M. Hillary, A. W. Lloyd and J. Swarbrick, *Drug Delivery and Targetting for Pharmacists and Pharmaceutical Scientists*, Taylor and Francis, 2001.

Index

Fundamentals of Medicinal Chemistry, Edited by Gareth Thomas
© 2003 John Wiley & Sons, Ltd
ISBN 0 470 84306 3 (Hbk), ISBN 0 470 84307 1 (pbk)

design for specific purposes, 197
improving absorption, 197
improving patients acceptance, 198
improving transport through membranes, 197
minimising side effects, 200
prontosil, 51, 195
site specific, 198–200
slow release, 198
tripartate prodrug, 196
Progesterone, 203, 204
Prokaryotes, 131, 132, 245
Proline, 2, 212
Propranolol, 169, 185
Prostaglandins, 141, 258
Prostaglandins synthase, 141
Prostanoic acid, 258
Prosthetic groups, 6
Proteins, 4–10
analysis, 9
anti-parallel β-pleated sheet, 8, 9
conformations, 6
conjugated, 6
C-terminal group, 5, 7
examples of the biological functions of, 4
fibrous, 8
globular, 8
glycoproteins, 6
haemoproteins, 6
α-helix, 8, 9
hydrogen bonding, 9
lipoproteins, 6
N-terminal group, 5, 7
order of structure, 8
parallel β-pleated sheet, 8, 9
peptide link, 4, 5
polypeptides, 5
primary structure, 7, 8
salt bridges, 8, 10
S-S bridges, 6, 7
secondary structure, 8–9
simple, 5
structure (general), 4–6
tertiary structure, 8
triple helix, 8, 9
water solubility, 9
Proflavine, 151
5-(Propnyl)uracil, 154
Protofibril, 9
Prunasin, 16

Pseudocholinesterases, 189
Pyranose, 11, 15
Pyrantel embonate, 63
2-(2-Pyridyl)ethylamine
Pyrrole, 108

Quantitative structure-activity relationship (QSAR), 40, 42, 78–91
Charton's steric parameter, 84
Craig plots, 88
electronic effects, 78, 81–83
Hammett σ constants, 78, 82–83, 84, 88
Hansch analysis, 85–88
Hansch equations, 86, 87
inductive constants, 83
lipophilicity, 78, 79–81,
lipophilicity substituent constant, 79, 80–81, 88
molar refractivity, 84–85
partition constants, 78, 79, 172
physicolchemical parameters, 78
regression constant, 81, 87, 253
steric effects, 83–85
standard deviation, 81, 87, 253–254
Swain and Lupton constants, 83
Taft M_s steric constants, 78, 83
Taft steric parameter, 84
Verloop's steric parameter, 84
quinine, 43, 151

Ranitidine, 40, 41, 168
Receptors, 41, 131, 132, 145, 147, 242, 247–249
β-adrenergic, 144
allosteric site, 146
domain, 247
down regulation, 38
drugs that target, 144–147
histamine, 144
ligands, 247
secondary messengers, 247
signal transduction, 247
superfamilies, 247, 248
Regression analysis, (see Quantative structure-activity relationships)
Resolution, 206, 207
Resting potentials, 246
Reverse transcriptases, 155, 156
5-(β-D-Ribofuranosyl)uracil, 16
Ribbonstructures, 99
Ribonuclease A, 10